Don't Wait Another Day Change Inside

Discover the Recipe to Your Whole, Big, Delicious Life

Catherine Hirsch

Printed in the United States of America.

Published by Author Academy Elite
PO Box 43, Powell, OH 43035
www.AuthorAcademyElite.com

Identifiers:
ISBN: 979-8-88583-207-6 (Paperback)
ISBN: 979-8-88583-208-3 (Hardback)
ISBN: 979-8-88583-209-0 (Ebook)

Library of Congress Control Number: 2023906446

Dedication

With love, to my dad (and all the men like him), my family,
my patients, and everyone who shares their whole, big,
delicious life with me

Table of Contents

Introduction

I remember the day I made a big shift away from the current medical model in America. Looking at my life now, it is hard to believe I have not always been a whole-food-plant-based-lifestyle-is-medicine kind of girl. I went to school to be a registered nurse, so for years, I was a medicine-is-medicine type. I have spent thousands of hours giving medicine and helping people to understand how their prescription medications work, but now my days and nights of passing medications are over. I came to realize I was not educating people on the most important thing, - lifestyle.

It started out as an ordinary day at work. My daughter called, but when I answered the phone, I could not understand anything she was saying—she was crying too hard. Every question I asked was met with more hysterical crying and incomprehensible words. Finally, I said, "Do I need to call 911? I can't understand you, and something is obviously very wrong. Do I need to call 911?"

To that, I got a howling emphatic, "No!" Looking back, I should have called 911. Not that her judgment was incorrect, but what if it had not been? Sometimes I am a little slow to hit the panic button.

I may not have hit the panic button, but as I drove home, I became more and more anxious, worrying and not knowing what I was going to find. When I got there, I discovered she had been in an accident, and her injuries included some broken bones. The next few months were quite an ordeal for her. At the same time, to me, it was a blessing that the accident was not worse. It was a wake-up call. That is when I decided that life is too short and unpredictable to waste another day being unhealthy and unhappy at work.

At that time, I was working as a telephonic case manager for one of the top five largest health insurance companies in the country. From a distance life was good—but the truth is I was middle-aged, putting on weight, and buying bigger sized clothes than I ever had before. I was not exactly the picture of health.

As I looked in the mirror and saw myself looking different on the outside, I was changing on the inside too. Most days I felt mentally exhausted. I had frequent headaches, sinus congestion, and my back hurt all the time. I did not pay much attention to these symptoms because I was busy with work and my family. In my mind, I reasoned that my changing health was because I sat at the computer all day and I was getting older. I figured my congestion was due to poor air quality where I lived.

My annual checkups showed my blood sugar level as borderline. To get a decent blood pressure reading, I had to sit without moving a muscle for twenty minutes beforehand. My cholesterol numbers were the worst they had ever been. Again, I was not alarmed by this because heart disease and diabetes were in my family and so I had an acceptance that it was only a matter of time before I would end up with those diseases. I took chronic diseases as something that was inevitable and was out of my control. I assumed part of getting older was being achier, putting on weight, and slowing down. My body was in constant overdrive, and it was beginning to catch up to me. It was like I was the head chef in a busy restaurant, but I did not take the time to choose what I was cooking. I thought it was normal to feel overloaded and stressed daily. That is what I heard others experiencing too.

Most of my friends and almost all my patients were experiencing the same decline in health. Despite spending lots of money on doctor visits, labs, procedures, and tests, the people around me were not getting healthier. In the span of 20 years in the medical field I was witnessing earlier onset of chronic diseases, more people debilitated and unable to work, and diseases such as obesity, type two diabetes, and fatty liver disease affecting younger people. What is the purpose of all the testing, procedures, and medications if the patients do not get better?

The burnout I was experiencing was, in part, because I was not taking care of *myself*. Just getting through the day felt like a chore. I began to take stock of my situation. I have since realized I was using my purpose of caring for others as an excuse to procrastinate on my own health. I was allowing American culture to dictate my health instead of me. I bought into the notion that I was destined for heart disease because it "runs in my family." I blamed my headaches and congestion on computer screen time and seasonal allergies. Besides, I "didn't have the money" to eat healthy all the time. Not only that, I felt like I didn't really know how to cook. I reasoned that being on the run with work and kids' activities made it pretty much impossible to have time to exercise and eat healthy. Those were some of the lies running through my head daily, keeping me in a negative headspace. One by one, I began to stop those thought patterns.

I had thought, *if I had more time*, everything would be okay. I kept thinking that when the kids were older I would l have more time to exercise and get healthy. Additionally, my financial health was in the same negative space. I was getting by, but not killing it. Trust me, I know how it feels to be upside down in debt. I am a mom of four and was living my life stressed out and over-extended. I thought if I worked hard, I would eventually have enough money to pay off the house, and then, I reasoned, I would not be as stressed and would be able to focus on my health.

We are often led to believe we are either in a positive headspace or a negative headspace. I think we can be in both, and that is what helped keep me stuck. I did, and do, have many positives in my life. I am productive at work, and I enjoy adventures and learning new things. I always have a project or two in progress. I have friends and family with whom I work and play. I always have something to do and people to see. I regularly volunteer at church, at school, and in the community. Despite what I put it through, my body was putting up with my neglect. While all those things were positive in my life, at the same time, I had those other negative thought patterns and stress compounding alongside the positive.

I wish I had been more proactive with my health earlier. I wish I had been more aware of how American culture and good marketing campaigns were influencing my behavior. I was ignoring the power I had within me to make decisions with a clear purpose instead of playing hot potato all day long. I did not recognize all the gifts available to me.

It would have been better if I had addressed my mindset sooner to minimize the negative and maximize the positive. I had goals and mantras, but I did not fully acknowledge the processes needed to go with them. So, even when I met my goals, success was quick to fade. I was still feeling poorly and bumping along financially. I failed to recognize the power in each moment of my daily routines to move me along in my journey. Spending money investing in myself did not seem like an option. Instead, I wasted a lot of time, money, and energy plugging away with the same old recipes that produced bland results.

These are the recipes that industry and government promote. Take supplements. Just be more active. Stay away from carbs and eat more protein. Do a cleanse. Join a gym. Get an activity tracking device. Believe me, I tried it all. The list goes on and on, keeping us spending money, chasing the latest new craze, and buying things we do not need. For me, lasting success did not come with any of those. The kicker is, I was a nurse and I *thought* I was taking care of myself! I *thought* I was avoiding what was obviously bad & did not abuse my body, but I was still experiencing a decline in health. I *thought* that as long as I limited unhealthy food and drink and consumed them only in moderation that I would be fine. Turns out, what I thought I *knew* was wrong.

Now I have processes—recipes—that work for me. Now I know what questions to ask to help move forward. I want to share them with anyone who is living life waiting for a better tomorrow. It was not until I made up my mind to seize on opportunities to make lifestyle changes and change how I thought about myself that I began to change my behaviors and see consistent progress. When I became dedicated to continuing that progress, I began to see lasting results in my health. The more I paid attention and appreciated how my daily life affected my BIG Picture, the easier it became to stay out of negativity loops. Not only that, but it has also improved my ability to help others with their health. This book is about how to make those changes. It works for me. It works for others. It can work for you too. Keep reading.

I quit my job within a few months of my daughter's accident. I had been disenchanted with my work for a while. I was helping people, but I knew I was not helping them with what was most important *to them*; I was helping them in ways that were most important for *the company*. Oh sure, I talked quite a bit with people about not smoking, diet, and exercise. Still, the real focus of medical care in America today, that most of my patient conversations revolved around, was centered on pharmaceuticals, medical procedures, testing, medical equipment, and surgeries, not lifestyle.

The world did not end when I quit. Instead, it became more joyful. Trading in being overloaded at work and overloaded with life was a game-changer for me. I had been afraid of jumping from the frying pan into the fire, but I needed to take the risk of changing my work and processes to move forward. That was when I began studying lifestyle—particularly nutrition, fitness, and mindset—more deeply.

I started to think: *What am I happy with in my life? What am I not satisfied with in my life? What changes can I make? How can I make my work more meaningful? What will make me healthy?* I was not going to wait until the kids were grown. I realized I had enough money. I made changes with how I spent my time. I did not want to keep living overwhelmed with endless activities and products that were not giving results or adding satisfaction to my life. I was not happy with my job, nor with how I was not taking care of myself. I was not pleased with the debt I had accumulated. I decided to rethink my routines to become a healthier me. I started making more decisions instead of thoughtlessly allowing others to make them for me.

The point is not that you should quit your job. The point is that we need to discover whether we are doing what interests us and moves us forward with our identity and purpose. In recognizing the power of how I speak to myself, I have made some obvious changes, such as moving from a suburban to a rural home and changing my work from hands-on nurse to a more remote coach and working outside. Most of my changes have been more subtle.

I researched the fascinating science of nutrition and fitness with books, articles, and videos. As I learned, I started putting the information into daily practice one piece at a time. I did not have it all figured out, but I knew there was something to lifestyle medicine that could help me and people I cared for who had chronic conditions. Initially, I was reading about small studies whose results seemed too good to be true, so of course, I had my doubts at first.

As I did more research, I became less skeptical and more partial to the concept of lifestyle as medicine. Lifestyle medicine is a natural place to start with preventative health. *Nutrition, activity, and stress management have long been known to impact health.* The hardest thing to process was that the conclusions the researchers reached were the opposite of what I had been taught and had been teaching about nutrition. Why hadn't I been taught these things in nursing school? That is another thing that was shocking. Much of the research is over fifty to one hundred years old! It is not new research!

My breakthrough was when I learned about the China project. It was huge and hard to ignore. I began to live and promote lifestyle medicine. I filled in knowledge gaps by becoming plant-based certified. I expanded my cooking skills with a plant-based culinary course and certificate. The more I grew into lifestyle medicine, the more I discovered credible doctors singing the lifestyle-is-medicine tune, all promoting the importance of good nutrition, exercise, relationships, and stress management.

Looking back, I wish I had learned more about lifestyle medicine sooner because it has been revolutionary for me. Focusing on mindset, practice, and community have made it easier for me to bounce back after setbacks and challenges. It shows in how I feel, and approach life and it shows in my numbers too. I have lost over 30 pounds, my blood pressure has improved, and my cholesterol numbers are the best they have ever been. I discovered a whole new world in lifestyle medicine.

In the process, it became clear how much our current medical practice lacks in promoting self-care. Instead, they prefer we bring our symptoms to them and trust in medications and procedures. Nurses do not practice health care. We practice sick care. The current popular culture of "recreational eating" and "fat-is-fabulous" is not helping either. Now I am healthy without exercising all day long and without counting calories, macronutrients, containers, points, or taking expensive supplements or medications. I have made being healthy a priority in my lifestyle, which has in turn given me more energy and appreciation for my community and the joys of life.

The notion that "fat-is-fabulous" is misguided. People are fabulous and people are more than their appearance. But overconsumption of fat is not healthy. Fat poses a risk to your body's health. The standard American diet is not aligned with health. It may be good for the health of the pockets of some, but over the long haul it is not healthy for Americans, our communities, or our planet.

If I had acted sooner, I would be further along, but life is not a race. I did what I could, with what I had when I had it. I cannot change the timing for me, but by spreading the message, I can change it for you and for others. After what I have learned through my research and my own lifestyle-is-medicine journey, I cannot go back to being a traditional registered nurse in the same capacity as I was before. Instead, it is more important to me to promote lifestyle medicine. I recognize the value of modern medicine and its advances. However, it is clear to me that much chronic disease could be avoided with a more significant focus on real prevention – not just screenings for disease. I believe people will benefit when they are empowered to be accountable for their lifestyle choices that impact their health. Focusing on prevention is accomplished with the recipe ingredients of nutrition, activity/fitness, mindset/stress management, and relationships. These ingredients can be used for *prevention* of disease, as well as for *intervention* of disease.

That is why *Don't Wait Another Day* is designed to give you the tools to embrace your big, delicious life starting the day you open chapter one. I will provide you with reasons why previous trends in health and wellness are flop recipes that create the poor health that is common in our communities today. I want to be clear about how best to use the time you have in a way that makes a difference for you and those in your life. I begin with helping you identify what is most important to you and why you value it. Creating a healthy lifestyle can be both attractive and satisfying because, when you are happy with your health, your mood improves, and so do your relationships. Some critics might say I am oversimplifying things. Well good. That is part of my goal. I believe good health does not need to be complicated.

At this point, you might be getting a bit anxious about exercising more because you do not like exercise. Maybe you hate the idea of spending time in the kitchen. Perhaps you are worried that your family and friends will not support lifestyle changes. Or maybe you just do not like vegetables. It is true there will be barriers, but we can work around them. If you are hesitant, read on.

I do not feel deprived when I rise out of bed in the morning to enjoy the day and make it count. I want that for you, too—if that is your desire. That does not mean every day has to be a flurry of production. It just means that we are not always waiting for "something" to happen before we get started growing in health and enjoying life more fully. I want *you* to feel in charge of your life—not your age, not your genes, not the government or industry, not your doctors, not your spouse or kids, and not just dumb luck. Choosing to take little life-enhancing actions creates healthy habits over time that leave us thankful for each day.

Then change snowballs. When we make ourselves healthy, we help our communities thrive. People are always watching us. We can be a positive influence. Some people get information and run with it, eager to share it with others. Some people keep information to themselves as if there is not enough health to go around, or perhaps to keep their competition down. I am one of those that believes everyone should have access to the information. Whether they use it or not is up to them. "You can lead a horse to water…" And maybe the horse will not drink. As I said earlier, using lifestyle as medicine runs counter to the current model in American medical care. Some will find it too strange.

Thank you for picking up this book. I hope that you are open to giving lifestyle medicine a chance, and you learn something new that you can add to your life to support your health. That openness will allow you to embrace lifestyle medicine to unlock its healing power. Put simply, lifestyle medicine means using day-to-day routines to promote health. Lifestyle medicine uses food, activity, and love to create health. That does not sound too weird, does it? I am here for you. Are you ready to get started?

This book is designed in three parts: Mindset/Imagine, Practice/Trust, and Community/Contribute. The first part has questions and action steps to assess where you are and get you moving forward to better health. I have thrown in some simple, 17 syllable recipes, affirmations, and mantras as well. You will walk away with a couple bonus Litmus Tests designed to help you make choices. These are simple questions you can ask to cut through the mixed messaging that is common in our culture. For this book, I want to focus on lifestyle choices and using these tests to tackle food addictions, stress, and activity addictions that suck up our time. Next, I bust some myths that held me back and may be holding you back too.

I want you to read aloud, write in this book, underline, highlight, fold down the pages—whatever it takes to use it and commit to your health. We each have our own learning style, and yet, most of us learn using some combination of all three techniques – visual, audio, and kinesthetic – so why not use all three to our advantage? The second part of this book is about putting healthy habits into action to prevent common, chronic diseases of western countries. Lastly, part three of this book covers how our health is part of our contribution to our community and how our environment shapes our beliefs. Our mental health, happiness, and satisfaction in life impacts those around us. We can use the truth found in five simple things to support our health as part of our contribution.

Most lifestyle medicine books go deep into *why* we should make lifestyle changes. I want to go deep into *how* to make lifestyle changes. It can all start today with your imagination. Picture what your body would feel like strong and healthy, believe it is possible, and consistently work toward it. They say Rome was not built in a day.

Or was it? I say it was.

Rome was built in a day—and a day, and a day, and a day.

I challenge you to do the same things with your health. Acknowledge your daily habits and why you do what you do. Choose to be dedicated to caring for yourself. This book will help you get clear with a plan, make sure your actions connect with the plan, cut through confusing health messaging, and stretch yourself to *grow* where you need to. I will be here for you whenever you need me. One day at a time, we can make choices with each other that turn into big results.

What we put our attention on grows stronger in our lives, so don't wait another day. Come as you are, bring an open mind, and change inside.

Discover the recipe for a big, delicious life!

What can you do today?

Don't wait another day to dive into Part Three!

PART 3

Community Contribute

"My life is my message."

-Ghandi

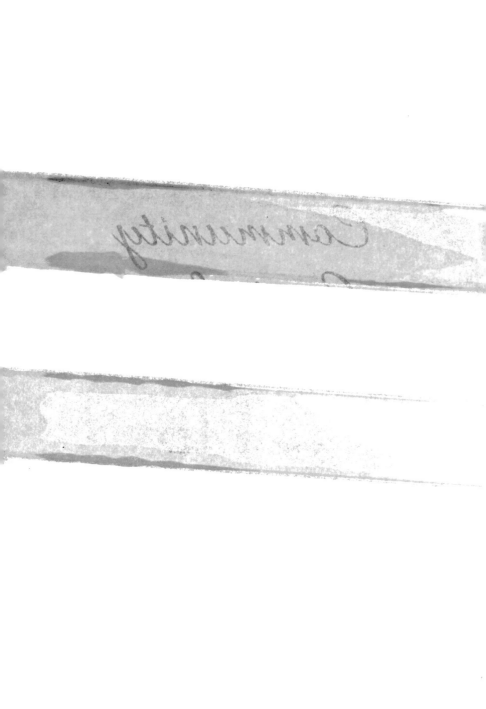
Community

CHAPTER TWELVE

System Failure

Considering the
Consequences down the road
I changed my lifestyle.

T he point of sharing some of my story through this book is to help reinforce the message that we oversee our own heath. Not only that, but it is our own responsibility. When we take care of ourselves, we are not burdening others with the consequences of our carelessness. If we could all understand a little more fully how our actions impact not only ourselves but others, we could cut back on a lot of pain and suffering.

Not to sound heartless. I know it is hard to hear. You must have the capacity to see that part of the reason you are unhealthy is your own fault. Few people or families want to accept that. It is not a person's fault that the system inherently confuses and misleads people, but it is up to individuals to find out the truth and know the truth. Sometimes we must hear it several times before it takes. If you have heard it repeatedly, see it, and choose not to act, that is on you, and it is to your own detriment. Industry is fine with this because you are supporting them by buying their products. The medical field is okay with his too because your illness keeps their industry thriving. Not being accountable for our own health does, however, have a negative financial consequence for society.

In my years of nursing, I have seen so much suffering in individuals and the grief it causes them and their families that it is hard to imagine not doing what we can to take care of ourselves. If you have been lucky enough never to have been touched by chronic disease or act as a caregiver, it may not interest you to help reduce the misery. Or maybe you think it is survival of the fittest – every man for himself. Keep in mind, when one man falls, we can all go down. The bell tolls for thee!

I want to help encourage people to be in charge of their own health, but I recognize some people may think, "*Who cares?*" Not too long ago, at the local market, I listened to an overweight, young man in his early twenties saying he did not care about taking care of his health. If he gets to do what he wants and dies at an early age from a heart attack, he reasoned that at least he enjoyed himself. I did not bother to interject anything into the conversation.

His statement already showed his recognition that he is doing what he prefers rather than choosing what is healthy. The attitude this young man has toward his health tells me he does not care much for himself, does not appreciate the body he has been given, and does not care about how his health might impact his family. Also, his statement reveals a common misconception that a person just has a heart attack and dies. This is childish and inaccurate, as more often, a heart attack is the beginning of years of declining health and disability.

I get it. When I was younger, despite being taught my body was a gift to be taken care of, there were times when I took my body for granted. I have not always taken care of myself. At times I have been downright reckless. As I spent time caring for others it only made sense to be more careful with myself. Even witnessing the inconvenience of minor injuries, like a sprained ankle or wrist, led me to a more careful mindset. As I have gotten older, I have gained a better appreciation of the human body as a magnificent work of art. I began to enter the age where I thought I was taking healthy actions, though I did not realize I was off track.

Sadly, both misguided paths (thinking, "*Who cares? I'm gonna have fun*" or trying to be healthy with inaccurate information) cost everyone through the burden of higher health care costs. According to The Atlantic it has been shown that the sickest five percent of the population consume well over half of the nation's total healthcare costs while the sickest one percent make up a fifth of healthcare expenses. The government takes money out of our paychecks to help cover the costs. Hospitals must accept anyone who shows up on their doorstep including both the uninformed careless and the hoodwinked, both of whom pass on the cost of preventable chronic diseases such as diabetes, heart disease, cancer, lung disease, and autoimmune disorders.

When I first met my husband, I remember talking about the fact that his insurance costs were higher because he was carrying the burden of some of his diabetic coworkers who seemingly did not bother to try to control their sugars, watch what they ate, or exercise. "Lifetime of Healthcare Costs" study from Synchrony shows premiums, out of pocket expenses, copays, and deductibles adding up to well over a quarter of a million dollars for the life of those with employee-sponsored health insurance plans. The cost is high for everyone and it is growing as drugs are subsidized and mandated. Medications do nothing to get at the root cause of disease which is often lifestyle. The documentary, "Code Blue," cites lifestyle as the cause in eighty percent of chronic disease.

The message that these chronic diseases are preventable with lifestyle choices is not adequately broadcast and what messaging is out there, is often distorted due to financial and political interests. There is too much to be lost by many if our current medical model were to help our population become healthier. The medical system makes money doing interventions and prescribing medications to people who are sick, not by keeping people healthy. The academic system continues to educate students on disease management rather than prevention because it benefits financially from industry support.

Therefore, the change required to create a healthier country is not going to come from the top down, from those currently running and benefiting from the system. It is not likely to come from the bottom up either because those who are impacted the most are least likely to be exposed to the truth about how lifestyle can create chronic disease. The change will come from responsible people in the middle squeeze who make changes in their lifestyles that help reduce the demand for healthcare and spread the message of lifestyle as medicine.

We in the medical field contradict ourselves, when over, and over, we site lack of exercise or lack of eating right in a patient's record. In the old days, the medical field often labeled these offenders as non-compliant. Now we are more politically correct in how we talk about them, but the medical field still sees it as individual failure. We offer patients very little accurate information on nutrition or exercise. We treat stress and anxiety with pills rather than lifestyle interventions. We have no problem trying to fix nutrition with a pill but offer scant support for eating good nutrition in the form of whole foods. It is not an individual failure. It is an education failure of the system due to a lack of education on what makes a person healthy. Doctors, nurses, therapists, and dieticians are just as confused about what makes a person healthy as the public because, as I said, the education system is corrupt.

Those with chronic disease are set up for failure by our current medical system. Those who work in healthcare are set up for failure by our current academic system. How can anyone eat the right foods when they are being taught the wrong information? How can we better manage and prevent disease when we are not clearly being taught the cause of disease or that we can treat, reverse, and prevent disease with lifestyle changes? I have heard Dr. Esselstyn repeatedly describe it as "unconscionable" that the medical system fails to provide lifestyle choices as treatment for heart disease.

I could not agree more. I would go as far as to call it a sin of omission, a form of lying. Of course, that only applies to people who know the information and do not share it. Withholding information that you know can solve a person's problem, because you deem them incapable of understanding and using the information, is not only dishonest, but also lazy. Retaining and controlling information because releasing it would potentially decrease revenue is even worse.

If you read my introduction, you already know the China project was an eye opener for me. It was enlightening not just into how the medical system works, but also how the academic system operates and how research findings are discredited by powerful influential industries when those industries feel the findings may threaten their profits. My questions about the medical system and ideas around lifestyle as medicine began before I learned of the China project so by the time I found it, I was already open to consider it and was looking beyond industry and media for answers.

The answers I have found are not popular, but they are **authentic**.

"

"And what do you benefit if you gain the whole world but lose your own soul? Is there anything worth more than your soul?"

Matthew 16:26

CHAPTER THIRTEEN

Loonatic Fringe

The loonatic fringe?
Or people seeking the truth?
There's no turning back.

In my search for clarity on nutrition, I found myself agreeing with a minority of physicians who promote whole food plant-based nutrition to support health and treat disease. I think of them as the loonatic fringe because media portrays their message as looney and unreasonable. The whole-food-plant-based message may be better received now than in the 1980's and 1990's, but, to me, it still appears fringe. My foray into the loonatic fringe questioning our food system and questioning our medical model had its foundation in three books. I did not read the books one after the other. There were books that I read in between over the course of a couple of years. I first read <u>Fast Food Nation: The Dark Side of the All-American Meal </u>by Eric Schlosser and <u>The Case Against Sugar</u> by Gary Taubes. I passed the point of no return when I read the last of the three: Dr. Caldwell Esselstyn's book, <u>Prevent and Reverse Heart Disease, The</u>

<u>Revolutionary, Scientifically Proven, Nutrition-Based Cure,</u> and saw the diagnostic pictures it contained.

I was excited the summer I read that last one. The day before we left for our Wisconsin vacation it arrived with other books I had ordered. I love to read. So, I usually take 2-3 books with me whenever I go on a trip. My excitement dissipated when I got into the first few chapters of Dr. Esselstyn's book. There I was in America's dairy land with cheese curds as far as the eye could see, and I was reading all about the benefits of not eating dairy. Not only that, Dr. Esselstyn was also recommending not eating anything that comes from a being that has eyes - this from a man who was raised on a farm with a family tradition of farming!

We were going to be fishing on our trip! What about all-you-can-eat Wednesday Night Chicken Wing Ding? What about Friday Night Walleye, and Tuesday Night Prime Rib Special? And no limburger cheese? What could I do? I enjoyed the vacation as planned, but with every meal and turn of the page I knew big changes needed to happen in my life on both personal and professional levels. Another of my vacation books that year was <u>The China Study Cookbook,</u> by Leanne Campbell PhD. One rainy day while I was reading it, my son looked over my shoulder at the Coconut Corn Chowder recipe and said, "Gross!"

(Of course, that was the first recipe I tried when we returned home.)

That was the beginning of easing more and more meatless days into my weeks which has now turned into years of meatless days. Now my meals are not always as put together as that corn chowder, but they all have a whole lot more flavor than they did before and a boatload more nutrition. Previously, the appeal of my cooking was in the salt and fat from the meat centerpiece. Now the appeal comes in the flavors of the food and spices: bean burgers, soups, salads, stir-fries, pasta, potatoes, burritos, tacos, spaghetti. On the surface it looks like what I was eating before, but much of the sugar, salt, and fat have been removed: hashbrowns, quesadillas, oatmeal, pumpkin pie, apple crisp, banana bread, potato salad, waffles, pudding, and fruit. I have learned to transform the recipes into health supporting foods.

After years of taking care of hospitalized heart patients, witnessing the life changing drama resulting from heart failure, heart attack, stroke, and kidney disease, then to read how the results of plant-based eating reversed disease in Dr. Esselstyn's group of end stage heart patients, led to a moment of epiphany. I have had an amazing career as a registered nurse in a variety of healthcare settings: hospital, homecare, hospice, long term care, health insurance, case management, and research. I already knew the system did not provide the results it promised. I witnessed firsthand over the years people becoming sicker at earlier ages. I already knew health organizations and non-profits were businesses which carefully craft their messages so as not to put off industry donors. Instead of giving clear messages about the impact of lifestyle on diseases such as cancer and heart disease, they continue to sit on the fence and give mixed messages.

When I read those three books I came with an inquisitive, open mind, curious for solutions. In their own way, each of the three books I previously mentioned brought clarity to how our current medical model works in America and how the food industry impacts our disease. I was gradually further waking up to how our food industry, medical practice, charitable organizations, politics, schools, and watchdog groups intertwine as I watched documentaries like, "What the Health?," "The Game Changers," and "Seaspiracy,"read more books, and took courses.

Along the way, I found out about the book The China Study Startling Implications for Diet, Weight Loss, and

Long-Term Health and learned more about its coauthors T. Colin Campbell, PhD and Thomas M. Campbell II, MD. I read T. Colin Campbell's book, Whole Rethinking the Science of Nutrition, and completed my plant-based nutrition certificate at T.Colin Campbell Center for Nutrition Studies and eCornell. I listened to his lectures about his China project, which took a close look at many dietary and lifestyle factors associated with disease in 170 villages in mainland China and Taiwan. A short while after that, I enrolled in the Rouxbe Online Culinary School and was conferred as a certified plant-based professional.

I was continually finding more doctors online in the world of lifestyle medicine like Dr. Neal Barnard, founder of Physicians Committee for Responsible Medicine, and his many projects such as the Food for Life program and the 21 Day Jumpstart. I also read Dr. Michael Greger's book, How Not to Die: Discover the Foods Scientifically Proven to Prevent and Reverse Disease and found his website nutrition-facts.org to be a smorgasbord of information on nutrition. Two of my favorites lifestyle doctors are Dr. Michael Klaper and Dr. Saray Stancic. The McDougall's, shed light on how old the information supporting lifestyle as medicine is, as Dr. McDougall pointed me in the direction of Dr. Pritikin, Dr. Kempner, and Dr. Swank. Mary McDougall has been inspirational in learning to cook healthy meals.

Another person who also fueled my quest for information on lifestyle medicine, was John Robbins through his book Diet for a New America How Your Food Choices Affect Your Health, Your Happiness, and the Future of Life on Earth and with his collaboration with his son Ocean Robbins on the Food Revolution Summit. "Plantpure Nation" was another documentary that implicated our cultural norms and political system in perpetuating our country's current state of poor health. I took note of the research done by Dr. Dean Ornish and that of the Framingham Heart Study.

Over the last several years, as I have absorbed information on lifestyle medicine, I have gotten better at cooking and eating clean by avoiding processed food as much as possible. Nutrition was just a part of the lifestyle changes I have made. On the fitness front I added running, swimming, roller skating, biking, kayaking, hiking, and walking more regularly into my days. I found fitness programs such as Beach Body and iFit helpful and have used yoga, and prayer to build a foundation for the rest of my lifestyle changes. I remain a work in progress. I am far from perfect, but I have come a long way.

I remembered a younger me, just out of nursing school, who said, "I think God has given us everything we need to be healthy in nature." What had happened to that girl? The seeker becomes the finder. I had been looking for her. I am glad to have found her again.

Part of why she got lost is because our culture portrays lifestyle medicine and its practice as radical. Many would consider those I have mentioned to be on the loonatic fringe. Looking at healthcare from a holistic point of view has been deemed too extreme. It is certainly not mainstream. Not once, in all my years of nursing, have I ever heard a doctor implicate a change in diet as cancer prevention or to treat multiple sclerosis. The doctors I work with may see the results poor diet causes on health, but they have not used it as first line treatment for disease. Long ago, when I attended a conference on using guided imagery as a non-pharmacologic technique for pain management, I remember the reaction I was met with when I took the idea to others, "*It sounds like you have joined a cult.*" At the time, I was not tenacious enough to remain looney.

I have newfound hope in lifestyle medicine and the loonatic fringe. A couple of years ago I gave someone my copy of The Engine Two Diet The Texas Firefighter's 28-Day

<u>Save-Your-Life Plan that Lowers Cholesterol and Burns Away the Pounds</u> by Rip Esselstyn. After a year or so, they returned it to me unread. Then about six months later they mentioned to me that their cardiologist had recommended the book as a resource.

The fringe is, at last, becoming less fringy. I walk in freedom as I **overcome**.

66

"You, dear children, are from God and
have overcome them, because the
One who is in you is greater than the
One who is in the world."

1 John 4:4

CHAPTER FOURTEEN

Take the Dubball

When we seek the truth
We find the light of the world.
Take that as a win!

I have not been brainwashed by the loonatic fringe. I have not joined a cult. I do not consider myself an activist. I am simply a person who has read a lot of books, looked at results of lots of research studies, watched, attended, listened to many lectures and podcasts, and lived over 25 years of my life as a registered nurse. All these things helped me to gather information about the impact of lifestyle on human health, animal health, and environmental health.

Any one of those three topics, or all of those, will often get people riled up. I have come to believe that the powers-that-be have purposely allowed division to be created around these topics. Public conversations around them have been so perverted that it is next to impossible to have a meaningful discussion about them. The impact of lifestyle on human health is my focus. Without health, so much of life's movement, productivity, and enjoyment is lost and replaced with suffering. This is ironic, being that the things people are led to believe create more enjoyment, end up leading to less satisfaction in the long run.

Research has shown that most people think things like money, health, and purposeful work create the happiness and satisfaction we want in our lives. We spend the bulk of our time chasing those. However, those are not the five things that most often are cited to contribute to happiness. Spoiler alert: money is not one of the five identified. The old saying "money can't buy love" exists for a reason. Often it is the opposite. Those with the most money are the least satisfied with life.

There is some overlap in the things in life that create satisfaction and the things that create health. In a way, our mental health is that feeling of being satisfied and happy with life. In order of least important to most important, the top five things that researchers have learned create happiness are: volunteering, exercise, sincere spiritual grounding, social connections, and, the most important thing, sleep.

If sleep is the most important, it is no wonder I was on the struggle bus for so long. I knew my lack of sleep was a problem, but I did not address it. Years of shift work, ever changing schedules, and raising children left me incredibly sleep deprived. At the time, I just accepted it as the way life is. Others around me were doing the same things. I could have done myself a favor years ago by sleeping more. (In part two of this book, I will go into ways to put boundaries around your sleep and make it a priority.)

Next in importance is social connections. Happy relationships with friends and family buffer the pains of life. Conversely, according to study, loneliness in the elderly can increase a person's odds of death. Loneliness is associated with less effective sleep, decreased immune function, and increased pain. If the pandemic taught us nothing else, it taught us that people, young or old, do not do as well in isolation. Prisons use isolation as disciplinary punishment because they know it is torment to be alone. Parents use time outs with toddlers. At a basic level we seek meaningful social contact with others. We can use this desire as a positive influence. As the saying goes… you can judge a man by the company he keeps. Surround yourself with those who share your values and together you will be stronger and happier.

The third thing that is associated with happiness or satisfaction is spiritual grounding. Spirituality gives meaning to the chaos of this world and can help a person look at the good, even in times of sadness. As a hospice nurse, I see this often in patients facing death. Believing in something bigger than themselves helps people cope better and sometimes even find joy in leaving this world for the next.

I will speak only for myself when I say time spent in sincere reflection and prayer at the beginning of a day gives me direction and at the end of the day helps to support my sleep. Improvement to mental and emotional health comes to the true believers regardless of what religion they practice. Daily habits of reflection often begin with awareness of self, others and the world, how our actions affect those things, and gratitude. For many this creates calmness and balance in their lives. This calming of the body can reduce stress levels leading to increased resilience and better coping.

Also, going to religious services can add to happiness because of the social connections made there. Spirituality is often grounded in love. Grace is this love put into action. This shows up as volunteering and supporting others in the community. Love is also present in loving the creator and receiving love and acceptance in return.

With spirituality comes the transcendence of knowing our identity beyond time and beyond the physical. Then we come to know and value truth, goodness, beauty, harmony, love, compassion, and joy. We begin to see our equality as we better understand the words of the Greek poet Horace who says, "only change my name and my story is also about you." We can begin to move away from fear of death and move toward greater meaning or our ultimate purpose in life. At times I am so distracted by the world around me that I fail to see the unseen. For me, when I am connected to God and the universe, the pain of separation and loneliness in the world is healed because I know I am never alone and I am loved.

Perhaps the most promoted thing of the five most important things that lead to happiness is the fourth, - exercise. Chemicals released when we exercise decrease stress and anxiety. These chemicals also boost our mood and brain function. Like spirituality, exercise can also be a social event and can release feelings of loneliness. High fives, laughter, camaraderie, and teamwork can go hand in hand with friendly, athletic competition. Like a church family, workout buddies can feel like family, give us a sense of belonging, and increase our happiness. Endorphins associated with happiness leave us feeling confident and capable of dealing with life. Yoga is an exercise that can help us become more connected to the earth, connected to our body, and connected to awareness that we are not just physical.

The last of the five things most associated with life satisfaction is volunteering. It makes people happy to know they are freely offering service for someone else for no reason other than that they want to. When I look back on times in my life I have struggled, I think of the people who helped me through. It inspires me to pay it forward and be that difference in someone else's time of need. Volunteering is an opportunity to take our personal transformations out into the world.

Volunteering does not have to be, but it is often interrelated with spirituality and social connections. Those who are more spiritual and socially connected often are generous with their time lending a hand to feed and clothe others, house people, care for the sick and the marginalized, or taking time to mentor or educate others. Be that as it may, at a basic level volunteering is being generous with our time. Acts of generosity, like exercise, have been shown to trigger the release of those feel good hormones: serotonin, dopamine, and oxytocin. This is part of what gives us those warm feelings of connection when we volunteer.

These five things are free for the taking: sleep, social connections, spiritual grounding, exercise, and volunteering. They are all connected in our life as a whole. Our natural impulses to love through connections of spirituality and volunteering and recouping with exercise and sleep support our mental health and happiness. Our culture attempts to hijack our happiness with fake relationships, fake food, fake education, fake medicine, fake news, all taking away our own well-being by taking those five things and the truth with it.

We are comfortable with the deception because the truth can hurt. It takes courage to listen to the truth, just as it takes courage to discern and stand up and speak the truth without fear of retribution. There is always a lamp at our feet to guide us and illuminate our way through the darkness. Without it we are helpless. To save ourselves and others we need to always search for the truth. Once we find the truth, our actions become the light of awareness for others.

We can begin again at any moment being a candle in the darkness. I mark that as a win. While it may relegate me to the fringe, I have learned to see and take the W's where I can. It allows me, even in times of uncertainty, to live a life full of **joy**.

21

66

"Therefore my heart is glad,
and my whole being rejoices;
my flesh also dwells secure."

Psalm 16:9

CHAPTER FIFTEEN

Living a Dream

A bizarre dream haunts.
As I wake to the next day,
Wait. What? It is real.

We experience the things we think about as if they are real. So, if we put our head in the sand and think about our own imagined reality does it become real? Apparently so for many. People surround themselves with those who will reinforce their false reality. It reminds me of the story of "The Emperor's New Clothes." This has been true for me practicing in our current medical system. I was surrounded by people who had been taught in the same system in which I was taught. So we all had the same ideas.

I am embarrassed to acknowledge how I used to view some lifestyle choices such as nutrition. For instance, I used to think of chicken nuggets, chicken patties, and Kentucky Fried Chicken as white meat, disregarding the high fat content of it. In the same way, my mind had been lulled into even considering pizza as healthy enough – with cheese as dairy providing calcium, sauce and veggie toppings for nutrients (ignoring any fatty meat toppings), and grains in the crust (never minding how refined and stripped of nutrition the grains were). It is sad to say that was how my mind worked in those days.

Only in removing myself from the typical way of thinking of food, did I discover how lifestyle, including whole food plant-based nutrition, can have a more significant positive impact on health. I have lost my career and identity in the medical system. What I have gained is improved personal health and comfort in knowing that lifestyle can help patients gain health rather than just help them to maintain whatever level of dysfunction they are at.

The last few years have opened my eyes to the extent of the manipulation of reality in the environment around us. I believe it is important to recognize how we are receiving information considering all the ways we are nudged to think a certain way. It is important to consider how we are being influenced whether we agree or not in an idea's truth. Our economies get propped up. Industry gets propped up with subsidies and bailouts. News stories pop up to distract or push certain agendas. Advertising bombards us on all sides. With all the deceit that surrounds us it is a constant burden which we all bear to determine the truth from the lies. This is important to recognize because technology plays a huge role in education both inside and outside of the classroom.

When the internet came out it looked like maybe it would help with that task of learning. Now it is doing the opposite as true information runs right beside false information. Search engine results, social media platforms, apps, and commerce platforms have the power to manipulate and censor information that gets seen. That is fine as long as users recognize the fallibility of the system and many users do not even consider it. Users also manipulate reality with filters and photoshop. Followers can be bought. Apps can automate engagement on what accounts like, follow, comment on, or unfollow.

The social media platforms are preying on our young. In example, the platforms can present content on eating disorders and negative body image to young girls in one location at the same time offering girls of the same age in another geographic area positive content. Minimum age is thirteen on some platforms but is easily bypassed as there is no vetting of the information used with new account set up. Many think the solution is not to give your kids a phone or change the minimum age. In my assessment that does not solve the problem. Parents would have to isolate their children from peers that have phones because they just borrow friends' phones. Social media is so pervasive and shape shifting in our society that parents have little control. Technology is always evolving and stays one step ahead of them. From Myspace, to Facebook, to Twitter, to Instagram, to Amazon, to Shopify, to Pinterest, to Snapchat, to Google, to Microsoft, to Indeed, to LinkedIn, to TikTok, and on and on - keeping up with how each one works is a full-time job.

The food industry has been around a lot longer than the internet and wrote the book on how to stay ahead of the crowd and target youth. With artificial flavors, colors, and additives much of our food is an elaborate illusion to appeal to our senses. Added sugar, salt, and oil help to make it addictive to our brains. Most of what is on our grocery store shelves is not natural. The food and its packaging are designed to manipulate us into buying it first based on how it looks and second on how it tastes. Nutrition is not really the selling points. Thank goodness for the ingredient labels! Labels do have wiggle room for deception, but at least they are there to give us a clue of how many artificial ingredients have been added.

More and more, however, there are plant-based products on the shelves. Their food packages *do* sometimes claim to be nutritious. They often use the use the same tricks to fool our senses. Plant-based cheeses, ice cream, and meats employ the same three little devils, - sugar, salt, and oil – that are what processed foods rely on. Now we have lab grown meat. It is expensive and inefficient to produce. The bottom line is many "healthy" or "vegan" alternative foods are not anymore real or healthy than the rest. One positive thing I can say about Beyond Meat and Impossible meat, is that they can act as transition foods as a person is moving toward eating more whole plant foods. Like manufactured "meat", meats that come from animals are also expensive and inefficient to produce. Without subsidies I wonder how the industry would fare. We are supporting a food industry that is making us sick.

Factory farms and slaughterhouses are tucked out of view from the general public. If we knew what went on, we might change how we eat knowing that beef was a living, breathing cow or calf, and that poultry was once a chick. We might choose differently if we realized that pig or that fish was sick with disease right before it was killed, processed, and sent to be bought and served on our plate. Millions of animals are "culled" in the farming process which is just a nice way of saying they were destroyed. We do not visit these factory farms or slaughterhouses to pick out the animal that we will eat for dinner like we might go to an orchard to pick apples or out to pick berries. We do not drive beside these places like we do crops. The fact that many of the crops we do drive by are for animals to eat, not humans, is also something that most people do not think about. The food system relies on reinforcing lies or misconceptions and hiding the facts. As I mentioned in the last chapter, it casts out those who object as if they are nuts or loons. It promotes the false notion that our bodies require only meat and animal products to provide protein.

You would think the medical field would step in and set people straight. You would be wrong. People do not realize inadequate care has become the norm in our hospitals, homes, and other facilities. Unless, they have experienced it directly.

In my experience, evidenced based medicine is becoming nothing more than lip service as science and evidence have become distorted by politics and the interests of big business. Expecting the leaders in our medical system to own the system's errors and the costs of medical mistakes is like waiting to hit a big lottery jackpot. Neither are likely to happen.

As terrible as it was, the pandemic was an opportunity to see our medical field through a different lens. I watched in disbelief as the powers that be isolated people and labeled some work non-essential, limited discussion regarding treatments, and shut down debate in general. I was surprised when vaccine mandates were announced and bribery, threats of job loss, and travel restrictions were used as forms of coercion to get the public to comply.

Post pandemic, I am still surprised, though not as much, with the lack of acknowledgement of reports of excess deaths in all age groups. I am dismayed by reports of thirty percent increase in heart attacks among our young people and I am stunned at the lack of discussion about over immunized people ending up with more infections. We have people getting paid to do incomplete research and then have a guaranteed market with drug mandates for their products and indemnity for any damage it may cause. Appallingly, the privacy our medical system claims to promote to protect a person, is now being overridden with everyone from our family to our bank teller, to the airline, to our employer feeling they have a right to know our vaccine status.

The experts continue to be propped up with an education system that is becoming less credible as industry interferes in it. It is not just higher education that is less credible. Our primary education is dubious as well. If it was easy to get passed as proficient in a brick-and-mortar classroom it is even easier online with plenty of ways to work around learning subject matter. The purpose of education is to gain knowledge of the truth. Instead, we are ignoring the truth and living in a land of illusion.

The world has become surreal for me to the point of being difficult to even put it into words. This much I can say, it is up to us to seek and follow the truth. Can we afford to bury the truth? How can we ignore technology automating what we experience? How can we ignore ultra-processed foods, monoculture crops, lab foods, fake meats, and more consolidated food production? How can we ignore the suffering of the sick, the declining, the disabled, the bedridden, and the incapacitated?

Is it all a dream? Was I just too busy working, raising a family, and trying to contribute to notice that all along I was being lied to and misled? I am sorry to admit that I did not see how badly medical education and research have been corrupted by the food and drug industries.

I am wide awake now with newfound **focus**.

"

"Look straight ahead,
and fix your eyes on
what lies before you."

Proverbs 4:25

PART 1

Mindset
Imagine

"The beginning is always today."

-Mary Shelley

CHAPTER ONE

Crush Cravings

> I eat in hiding.
> Craving exhilaration,
> I sneak to find more.

H ave you ever eaten until you were ready to burst? Guilty as charged here. Have you ever noticed there are foods you just cannot stop eating? I have. I used to be a regular Cookie Monster. Some foods are addictive. We crave these foods, and we overindulge on them. This affects our health and often our relationships. Those that make processed foods are aware of the addictive power of sugar, oil, and salt and they use it to their advantage. Their products are created with the purpose of cashing in on our addicted brains. They hire people for the specific role of making their products addictive. Our culture is soaked with messages urging us to eat unhealthy foods, drink unhealthy drinks, and then take medications to reverse the damage caused by those foods and drinks.

The messages come in advertising on the radio, on billboards, in newspapers, magazines, television, and our phones.

It is a never-ending deluge. It is not just advertising; the directive is also in many everyday activities too. Watch a ballgame? You will be encouraged to eat hot dogs, burgers, and beer. Then you will see ads for this, that, and the other pharmaceutical. Go to the movies? You will be served popcorn, candy, and soda. Grabbing a bite to eat? You will get fried anything and everything. The marketing claims any damage you do, can be undone by the wonderful medications your doctor can prescribe (pay no attention to the fine print or Mach speed verbiage at the end of the ad).

As a nurse, it is impossible to ignore addictions in America. It seemed every night I worked I had someone going through detox from either drugs or alcohol in my care. It was not uncommon to have another one or two patients in my group being watched for symptoms to set in. I am not a person who carries a ton of work stories in my memory, but one I *do* remember is of a thirtyish man transferred to me in the ICU from one of the floors. Upon transfer we had an order for leather restraints (one step away from being put on a ventilator with sedation). As we were struggling with him, he made a make-believe pistol with his thumb and index finger and said, "Bang, bang, bang, bang, bang, bang, click." Then he put the gun down and resigned himself, giving us an opportunity to get him under control.

The fact that even in his delirium he knew he ran out of imaginary ammunition was funny, but other than that, the whole situation still saddens me. I prefer to push the deaths I have witnessed caused by liver failure or bleeding out from esophageal varices out of my mind as much as possible, but the memories are there as evidence of addiction around me. Witnessing the suffering of so many patients makes it hard to forget.

I think food addiction in America is overlooked because it is a quieter disease. It looks tame in comparison to drugs and alcohol addiction. We do not have to wrestle with 300-pound people to get them to stay in bed. We may have to wrestle to *move* them in bed or get them *out* of bed, but overweight patients, unlike many of those suffering from substance abuse, do not try to attack you. The lack of belligerence and combativeness makes the addiction less obvious.

Do not let its quiet nature fool you. We know obesity is linked to many chronic diseases. Excess weight changes how our body moves, putting extra strain on muscles and joints. Carrying extra weight makes us short of breath even with simple activities like walking. Everyone is unique, beautiful, and valuable. Size is not the issue. The issue is that fat in our blood and in our organs is not healthy. Those who liken addressing obesity to fat shaming or portray fat as fabulous are making the problem worse. It benefits their profits for people to remain indifferent or proud of being overweight. So, they try to sell that line. For many people, as they put on weight, they begin to change their identity and how they see themselves. Over time they begin to put limits, consciously or unconsciously, on what they believe they can do.

You do not have to rely on someone else to give you statistics telling you the American population is heavier. It is apparent at the mall, at the movies, at a concert, in restaurants, at the grocery store, and at sporting events. Look around and you can see people are gaining more weight and they are gaining it at younger ages. As a result, the medical cost of obesity and its related diseases is growing too. In the recent coronavirus pandemic, we have seen how obesity affects the body's response to viruses as well. Poor health and addictions place a burden not just on individuals, but on families, communities, and the country - as we have also seen with the recent pandemic.

People are confused about what to eat when there is no need to be. This is what that confusion often sounds like.

I received this text from a woman I was talking with about weight loss. "There are so many different thoughts out there. All plants, no carbs, all protein. Who do you listen to? We will just do what we think is correct. You have to balance carbs and proteins and everything else. With so many different thoughts out there, they can't all be correct. So you take from all the ideas." She ended up going on a "sugar-free diet" recommended by a therapist because she could not wrap her head around not eating meat and dairy, which as you will discover in part-two, is a core ingredient in my recipe for health.

In one of our last conversations she said, "No. We will eat meat, poultry, fish, eggs, and cheese. The only thing processed is the cheese." At least she got the message of looking for less processed foods. Though we are not working together anymore on her weight-loss, she still occasionally sends me recipes for feedback on. The ingredients are sometimes using good whole foods. Often the problem is, the recipes call for ½ to one cup of olive oil or butter (sometimes more or both!). In her mind, oil, butter, and cheese are processed, but okay for health.

The confusion is in large part due to the food industry pushing processed foods which are made of plant fragments using refined sugar, oil, and refined flour. These fragments are vegan, but certainly not whole foods and they lack nutrients because their original fiber, vitamins, and minerals have been taken away. What is more, packaged foods are designed to be addictive made up mostly of fat and refined carbohydrates. This is why we crave foods that are bad for our health even though we know they are not healthy. Processed foods trick our brains by exciting it with artificial ingredients. Manufacturers further rely on these fake ingredients including preservatives, dyes, and flavors to give them a long shelf life while maintaining their colors.

The confusion and deception promoted by the food industry is not new in American culture. Over one hundred years ago Upton Sinclair was writing about it in his famous novel, *The Jungle.* "How could they know that the pale-blue milk that they bought around the corner was watered, and doctored with formaldehyde besides? When the children were not well at home, Teta Elzbieta would gather herbs and cure them; now she was obliged to go to the drugstore and buy extracts – and how was she to know that they were all adulterated? How could they find out that their tea and coffee, their sugar and flour, had been doctored; that their canned peas had been colored with copper salts, and their fruit jams with aniline dyes? And even if they had known it, what good would it have done them, since there was no place within miles of them where any other sort was to be had?"

I was told in school that this novel changed industry but look at the ingredients listed on the nutrition label on product after product. You will see chemicals that you probably cannot identify. I cannot even pronounce them, let alone know what they are and how they are made. Finally, I have learned that if I cannot pronounce it, I do not need to eat it. Furthermore, the meat industry does not seem to be better off than it was one hundred years ago. In some ways, it may be worse. Documentaries show current practices that are cruel and unsanitary sometimes leading to what the National Institute of Health refers to as "humane" large scale euthanasia to dispose of diseased animals.

It is not secret that I have my struggles with addiction. I would say that most people do whether they care to admit it or not. We are led by our culture straight to caffeine, chocolate, coffee, sugary pops, candy, beer, wine, alcohol, and prescription drugs. Our brains are wired to seek out pleasure and avoid pain and these things may all offer temporary relief or pleasure. Now I clearly recognize the power of addiction on my brain, and I purposely make decisions to avoid my weaknesses as much as possible. Not only that, I set up barriers to make it harder for me to be trapped by addiction. You can too. It may not work one hundred percent of the time, but for me, it is close. Alcohol and processed foods no longer seem as attractive when I consider long-term wholeness and joy in my life. Coffee has proved to be the hardest for me to quit, but I have cut back immensely choosing instead to drink decaf or caffeine free herbal teas.

It seems like I have been surrounded by alcohol since I was a teenager. It was always available. Often people who were overindulging invited me along for the ride. In that regard, being a young mom saved me because thankfully I recognized taking care of young children is best done when not impaired. Unfortunately, I fell for the rational that, in moderation, alcohol is nothing to worry about.

The crazy thing about alcohol is that cultures continue to promote it despite knowing it is not our friend. I often hear things like, "I only drink socially." Okay. That does not change the fact that alcohol impairs our decision making leading to more accidents, danger, and recklessness. Not only that, it leads to poor dietary choices. Ever notice how much junk food you crave when you drink? Also, alcohol itself is empty calories with no nutrition. It inhibits our ability to burn fat – some estimate up to thirty percent! It is a known toxin to multiple organs including our liver, brain, heart, and kidneys. Not to mention it is listed as a known carcinogen by both the U.S. Department of Health and Human Services as well as the World Health Organization (realizing that at this point the credibility and integrity of these organizations is questionable).

Think about that. We spend millions on cancer research. At the same time, we mass produce and promote what is known to cause cancer. What sense does that make?

In comparison to alcohol, ice cream and cheese seem harmless. Though they are not. They are addictive for me too and over time can cause serious health problems. I pay attention and plan for when I know I will be around them. This is almost all the time because our society is literally cheese and dairy filled. Once I began to recognize how our American culture has prescribed these addictive pleasures I began to *choose not to be hooked.*

I choose not to have the chronic sinus congestion dairy has caused me for years. I choose to breathe freely through my nose. If sinus congestion is a problem for you, I whole-heartedly recommend cutting dairy for 2-3 weeks and see if you notice a difference in how you feel. Cheese, yogurt, sour cream, milk, - the works- skip the whole section. You will likely notice weight loss and money savings as well. Also, I choose not to increase my risk for heart disease or cancer. I could go on, but you probably get my point. We have choices.

The reality I have witnessed with my own eyes and ears is that people who have addictions are not alone. If we are honest, most everyone does. Some addictions are less obvious and more socially acceptable. Workaholics, those obsessed with a particular hobby or sport, and those addicted to making money tend to be admired. Nevertheless, even behavioral addictions have effects on our health, which over time can be destructive. You might scoff, "*Really, what is the harm of being addicted to social media? A little scrolling never hurt no one.*" Be careful. What pops up next is curated especially for you and your history on that device. Are you in the group that gets messaging on alcohol, eating disorders, or suicide? Or have you managed to land in the group that gets magic eye pictures, or seemingly benign quizzes?

Be it the food industry, big tech, or pharmaceutical & chemicals, corporations have managed to have themselves recognized as individuals. They are addicted to making money regardless of the cost to others. Then they escape account-ability and blame the addict. Just as a typical addict blames others for their choices. Profits are their priority, their choice, not the well-being of their consumers. This makes your health and safety your responsibility.

For instance, people accept that cigarettes can be addic-tive. What makes them so powerful? Yes, the nicotine, but that is not all. Manufacturers add sugar as well. It is added in for a purpose. Is it to make them taste better? Maybe. Is it to make the addiction more powerful? Perhaps.

Compared to cigarettes and alcohol we are lulled into thinking food is not as harmful. Again, we are encouraged to use the idea of moderation when we eat. While we can easily see that the tobacco industry cashes in on our addiction, we do not clearly see that the food industry is doing the same thing. Like cigarettes, processed foods rely on the addictive power of sugar. Fatty products (including animal meat) can also be addictive. Think you will switch to processed plant-based options? Perhaps not, they are using the same old tricks in these processed foods as well. Dairy products have not only sugar and fat but digesting the protein in dairy can produce morphine-like compounds that attach in our brain to keep us coming back for more. This same protein in dairy has also been shown to promote cancer growth. Proteins in dairy are also suspect in Type 1 diabetes. Like cigarettes and alcohol, our food addictions *do* have serious consequences beyond just changing our appearance.

Have you ever eaten a pint of ice cream in one sitting? Been there. Done that. Those ingredients are part of the reason for that. It is not just about will power and knowing when to say when. It is about the brain craving and seeking sugar and fat-filled foods.

Salt is another highly addictive taste that manufacturers use to their advantage. Have you ever eaten the salt crumbs from the bottom of the potato chip bag? Yep. You are not alone. Manufacturers create junk food with the purpose of addicting people to it, so they have repeat customers, repeat customers, repeat customers. Should I say it again? Repeat customers.

Like the manufacturers, restaurant chains are aware of the power of food addictions. "Would you like some extra cheese on that?" might not be as innocent a question as you think. The United States government and its various health agencies are aware of the power of addiction. Your tax dollars help pay for the research, but unless you look independently, you are not getting a clear message of what the research results are. Put simply, the desire for a good economy and the power of industry lobbying leaves the message from the experts watered down and misleading.

Do these contradictions sound familiar? Eat less fat but get your dairy. Eat less fat but eat chicken. Watch your cholesterol but eat eggs and meat.

What if instead of putting their effort into making food addictive, the food industry switched gears and put more effort into making food as nutritious as possible? Isn't the real purpose of eating to fuel our body? The good news is, we can make that change ourselves. We can *choose* to put nutritious whole food in our body rather than processed foods that come in brightly packaged bags and boxes with cute fonts and logos. We all know the more you eat unhealthy foods, the more likely you are to become unhealthy. I have witnessed it firsthand for the past 25 years though in the beginning I did not clearly recognize the problem.

We can use food to protect ourselves from chronic disease and infectious viruses and bacteria. We have the power to eliminate the oxidative stress in our bodies that is cause by free radicals by eating antioxidants only found in plants that are provided naturally to us from above (or from the planet, or the universe – however you like to think of it). When free radicals outnumber antioxidants, it leads to oxidative stress and disease such as cancer, stroke, heart disease, multiple sclerosis, Parkinson's, respiratory disease, and others. When we see that our actions – what we eat and what we do – affects our health, we put ourselves in charge, - not doctors, not industry, not the government. Eat more healthy nutritious foods and you will become lean and healthy.

Most of us can recognize that eating cookies, cake, and potato chips are not healthy choices. Yep. We know that sausage, cheese, and bacon are full of fat. Duh. These processed foods increase damaging free radicals in our body. So, flip it. When we eat nutritious foods, we are supporting our health. We do not all need a science degree to figure it out or a government department or world agency to direct us.

We can place ourselves in charge. At the same moment, we are obeying biological laws of health that were given to us since the beginning of our time. Simple, natural food has been shown to be healthy over and over. We protect our bodies when we eat healthy food and avoid added chemicals. We support our health when we exercise and take time for movement. We support our immune system when we limit the input and stress our culture puts on our life. These are basic truths that we do not need science or double-blind studies to back up.

We protect our bodies when we eat healthy food and avoid added chemicals.

I remember 30 years ago saying I believed we have been given everything we need to be healthy in nature. I was a firm believer in music, pet, and alternative therapies like healing touch and guided imagery. Yet for years I was swept away from those ideas working in hospitals that make incredibly little effort to incorporate those methods of treatment.

We can choose to move toward eating a rainbow of whole plant-based foods. These are the foods our bodies were designed for and function most efficiently on. Plant foods are the only whole food that contain fiber. In fact, plants are high in fiber, low in fat, and contain no cholesterol. Plant foods are filled with antioxidants that boost our immune system so we can fight off disease and infection.

Whole plant foods are full of nutrients, vitamins, and minerals: calcium, beta-carotene, lycopene, vitamin E, vitamin A, selenium, phytochemicals, zinc, potassium, and countless more! Plants are the only foods that contain the antioxidants that fight free radicals. Animal products do not contain antioxidants. Foods like sweet potatoes and berries are good sources of antioxidants. Garlic is another plant-food with antioxidants and antimicrobial and antiviral effects. Even if you prefer to continue eating animal products, you can add more of these plant foods to your diet.

Plant fiber fills us up. How many times have you stuffed yourself on apples or carrots? This kind of over-stuffing does not happen because the fiber in plants helps us feel satisfied before we can overeat them. Fiber is also important because it absorbs unwanted toxins, hormones, and other chemical wastes and carries them out of our body. Without fiber, those things go back into our bloodstream and can make us sick. Unfortunately, the average American eats less than half of the recommended goal for fiber intake. It bears repeating, plants are the only foods that contain fiber.

It is worth the effort to move away from animal foods and processed foods if you truly want to regenerate your health. Typical Americans eat only about ten grams of fiber a day. A plant-based diet will easily provide three to four times that amount which is what is recommended for health.

As industry constantly goads us to eat and do what is unhealthy, we must hold onto hope, be mindful, and trust ourselves to make thoughtful decisions. Hope never stops.

"Hope"
by Emily Dickinson

Hope is the thing with feathers -
That perches in the soul -
And sings the tune without the words -
And never stops - at all —

And sweetest - in the gale - is heard -
And sore must be the storm -
That could abash the little Bird
That kept so many warm -

I've heard it in the chillest land -
And on the strangest Sea -
Yet - never - in Extremity,
It asked a crumb - of me.

While hope helps us move forward, it is not enough to hold onto hope that the world will change. It is our love inspired actions that will change the world. We must act by changing our behaviors to obtain the healthy life we desire and were made for. It is up to us to be aware of our tendency toward addictions and how others attempt to influence our behaviors. It helps to also remember that behaviors can be addictive too: shopping, work, a hobby, sex, social media, television, even exercise. Any of these can suck up our time, leaving less opportunity to build healthier habits and leaving less opportunity to celebrate the glory around us and enjoy our life.

Focusing on where to place blame for health problems does not solve problems, but it is helpful to acknowledge the source of the mixed messaging to figure out how we can avoid the pitfalls around us. Fighting darkness only creates more darkness. Instead, we can choose to override outside influences and recognize our own ability to impact our health. Ask yourself, *what are you hoping for?* When we recognize what we are hoping for it helps us be the light of awareness and be born again as we decide where to put our time and commitment and what things to let go of.

Whenever I work with someone who wants to break an addiction, we discuss why, when, and how they are going to quit. Planning for quitting an addiction is a lot like cooking. Before you even begin to cook, you must decide what you want to make, considering flavor, nutrition, and your skills. Then gather the information, ingredients, and equipment needed. Good planning involves deciding and gathering; however, the first step is always the decision.

The decision is the challenge. Everybody has 24 hours a day. Everybody can choose to behave in a way that moves them forward. To change, you have to challenge yourself by making the decision. Anyone can make that decision. Anyone can start fresh.

For smokers, I ask them what triggers their desire to smoke. Also, if they quit, what are they going to do with their hands? Putting thought into knowing what triggers our addictions and planning to gather replacement activities can make it easier to kick any habit.

Whether forming a healthy habit or breaking an unwanted habit, the *what*, the *when*, and the *where* are important decisions to get the desire out of our heads and onto the calendar. As they say, "What gets scheduled gets done." Then we start planning. This can make all the difference in how we deal with addictive foods and activities when we encounter them. Part of this planning includes deciding what healthy habits we could use to replace our unhealthy habits or addictions.

What are some healthy habits you have? As you identify them say them aloud. Acknowledge your good.

_____

_____

_____

_____

What are some healthy habits you would like to improve on or begin? Go ahead and write them down. We will use these later to stack on new healthy habits.

_____

_____

_____

_____

We can replace unhealthy habits or addictions with healthy ones, consider for a moment any addictions you may have.

You can list them here:

_____

_____

_____

_____

Thinking of any addictions you identified above, ask yourself why you would consider quitting and then if you find your reasons convincing and are ready to move beyond consideration, - when are you going to quit?

Write down the date along with any triggers you can identify. Start thinking about other ways to deal with your triggers. Are there any constructive activities that could replace your unhealthy habit?

Why?

_____

_____

_____

Quit Date:

_____

_____

_____

Triggers

_____

_____

_____

Replacement Activities

_____

_____

_____

We also must plan for symptoms of withdrawal. For instance, if we cut back on sugar, we know we might get headaches, feel anxious, restless, or irritable (sounds like withdrawal from cigarettes, doesn't it?). A plan might sound something like this: if I get a headache I put a cool cloth on my head and lay down for ten minutes. Or it could be this: if I start to feel restless, I will go outside and take some deep breaths and a short walk.

If you feel your symptoms may be severe, a visit to your doctor to consider medications is advisable. I should also mention that if you are currently taking multiple medications, it would be helpful to seek a doctor who is supportive of lifestyle medicine and let them know you are making changes so they can make dose adjustments as needed. Medications for heart disease, blood pressure, diabetes, or other chronic conditions will likely be decreased if not discontinued altogether.

Becoming aware of our habits and addictions gives us a starting point. From there we can imagine where we want our progress to take us. Know that as we start this process the goal is not merely to get us to the end. We are always growing. We just need faith that we will be granted things not yet seen that will help us on the journey. Faith is believing without seeing or without evidence.

How do you want to spend the rest of your life? In declining health and disability? Or active and capable doing activities and work you enjoy?

If you have not answered or thought about the questions posed so far in this book, go back, and fill in the blanks (or at least go back and sit with the questions as you consider the answers).

Next, when you go to bed tonight, I want you to notice your bedtime routine.

First, I....

_____

_____

Then, I...

_____

_____

When you wake up tomorrow morning, I want you to do the same thing. What is your morning routine?

First, I....

_____

_____

Then, I...

_____

_____

Chilled, sliced, strawberries
On warm toast with applesauce -
Simply delicious!

Read the next line aloud.

I have faith health is in me.

Read and repeat, as often as necessary.

Do not underestimate the power of the spoken word.
Speak the words out loud and move forward in health.
Consider writing it on a card and placing it
where you see it often.

I have heard it said that deaths caused by the medical system
is the third leading cause of death. I am not sure how that
statement is supported, but I can tell you from experience
that traditional medical practice in America did not improve
my declining health.

CHAPTER TWO

Take Heart

It begins when you
Make magic by starting fresh
Right where you are at

Once you have made that Decision (with a capital D) it is important to have the start date. When are you going to start making changes? I say why not today. Big changes can start small. Or big changes can start big, either way, - your choice. Start getting your plan together by assessing where you are at and addressing your mindset.

I am sure you have heard how important a positive mindset can be. You may have also heard that humans are hardwired for survival with a negative mindset that is motivated by things like fear and scarcity. To achieve a positive mind, we have to learn to overcome some of our natural focus on the negative. To do this, it is easier to learn to become less negative than trying to be more positive. In other words, it is easier to keep our thoughts and what we say more in the middle ground.

When people tell us to look at the positive or the silver lining after something bad has happened, it may seem like we are lying to ourselves because we are ignoring the reality of the negative event. It may feel like we are not being authentic or honest with ourselves about how we are feeling. Always searching for the silver lining can be helpful, but it is harder because of this inner conflict. It can help to think about what we can do to help work through sadness or anger in the moment. Sometimes when we do these things it leads us to seeing a possible positive perspective. Instead of us finding it, the silver lining finds us. Then we are able to reframe negative events, visualize success, and develop a plan of action.

What do you do when you are upset? Break things? Hit something? Yell? Take a walk? A run? Play an instrument? Sing a song? Deep breathing? Go outside? Pound on the piano? Drink a glass of water? A cup of tea? Talk to someone?

When we work through emotions by talking to someone, we can learn to become less negative by controlling our language. When we say something out loud, we give it more power than if we are just thinking it. If we do not give an idea power by verbalizing it, then we are less likely to act on it. Controlling what we say is a powerful way to cut back on negative thoughts. Sometimes venting negative ideas just makes our mindset more depressing, and at the same time (unless we are venting to a pillow), it affects those to whom we are talking.

It can be okay to vent, but I believe it is important to give yourself a timeframe and be more prudent about who you are venting to. Say you did not get a promotion you were aiming for or you did not get picked to be a team captain. Talking about it, blaming others, and talking garbage about the person who did get promoted or nominated does not change the result and it does not move you forward either. The more you rant or vent about it the more it brings the whole team down. Say what you have to say, gather any positives, and move on.

Try not to be a negative pull on the same person (or group of friends) day in and day out. Are you talking with someone who will be objective? Someone who can offer perspective? Dwelling on the past mistakes and failures of ourselves and others by talking about it out loud externalizes negativity in our life and gives it more power. In effect we get stuck in a negativity loop (and anyone else we bring on board to hold hostage in our loop). These negativity loops have potential to build stress in our mind and that of those we share it with. So do not randomly dump your stuff on people you do not even know or someone else who is already under stress. Use a little care.

To say the spoken word is more powerful than our thoughts is not to say thoughts and feelings are not important. Beside changing what we say aloud, we also must change what we allow ourselves to dwell on internally. Stopping negative thinking is a good strategy to become more neutral. When I find myself replaying a negative event or conversation, I tell myself, "*Stop. It's done. Don't think about it anymore.*" Depending on the event, this might take a few days to a week to get it out of my head. Sometimes after a code or death at the hospital I would get stuck replaying the day in my head. At first it could be helpful, but there would come a point when replaying it was stirring up more negative emotion in me than any positive gain. It did not do anyone any favors by talking it over either.

This is where prayer or meditation can be powerful. Offer your troubles up and have faith they will be sorted out. You get the release without adding to someone else's plate.

Ruminating on past negative events or failures does not have a place in moving forward in a positive manner. We can train our mind to notice our negative thoughts and try shifting our attention to something positive instead. It takes practice, but the more we pay attention and are on the lookout for these negative loops the easier it is to reset.

With that in mind, it is also important to be aware of who is feeding us negativity externally. If you have negative people who vent to you it is important to not let their negativity bring you down. This is also important to keep in mind when watching the news, watching movies or television shows, reading books, playing video games, and listening to the radio. So many of these media sources are there to benefit themselves by keeping us consuming their product. Lots of the time they promote what helps them and their investors and advertisers, not what is good for people as individuals. I always tell my kids to be careful what they put in their heads because once you let it in, you cannot get it out.

I was in my twenties before I started learning to step back. It took another 25 years before I got good at it. A few rules of thumb for me are to try not to say every negative thing I think out loud. Limit negative intake. Once I have observed anything helpful, I leave the past behind. Observation means learning to step back and see the situation rather than get carried away with emotion. This has been a lifesaver. Deep breathing is another tool that works wonders. I was with a patient and her husband not too long ago and he said over time they learned "lots of problems work themselves out." Offer it up and have a little faith.

This is where I was at when I started making changes. I was a registered nurse who had not received adequate training in lifestyle methods for exercise, nutrition, and stress management in nursing school. I was "too busy" with family and work to pay attention to the decline in nutrition my family and I was eating. I was spending more time sitting in the car and sitting at a computer or phone. In addition, my blood pressure was elevated, and my fasting blood sugar was rising. My weight was going up too.

Have you ever noticed your pants do not button as easily? My clothes were my first clue that things were amiss. Similarly, clothes can be testament to weight loss. One of the women I coached on creating healthy lifestyle habits said it best, "I put on a pair of pants today that I had not worn in a couple of weeks and could not leave the house until I found my belt."

Is your blood pressure elevated or your fasting blood sugar rising? Your doctor may not say anything about it, but you have been at all your appointments, and *you* know. Without even reading your chart you know 138/84 is higher than the last time you had it taken. Fat, sugar, decreased activity, and lack of fiber can all add to a slow steady weight gain that can creep up on us. We are conditioned to accept it as part of aging. Excess body fat challenges our body's function and performance. It also changes how we identify with ourselves.

That was my experience. Sometimes I would take my blood pressure at the automated machine in the grocery store and notice the numbers creeping up. My blood sugar was rising, and my cholesterol numbers were elevated. My weight was going up too. But at my appointments nothing was ever said about changing my lifestyle. Sometimes they might say, "You're borderline. Come back in 3 months so we can keep an eye on it and reevaluate." I began to accept that I was on the road to needing blood pressure medicine and maybe diabetes.

The problem is that until you have a disease, you do not get health care. No effort was ever put into educating me about lifestyle choices that were affecting my health. For a long time, I did not question the mixed messages I was getting. I did not question the sources and how they were affecting my mindset. There is a lot of talk about preventative medicine, but really what is called prevention is just monitoring, being influenced to comply to screenings with fear of surgeries or a pillbox crammed full of medications. Chronic disease can be treated better with lifestyle changes rather than medications and procedures because when we change our lifestyle, we are stopping the repeat daily injury of a bad diet and a stressful, sedentary life.

A mom whose daughter I recently coached describes it, "You've really been a lifeline here. The doc left me with "change her diet" instructions and nothing else. They really left us empty handed with no guidance at all. I can see how people have a hard time. You've made a world of difference giving us tools we need to really succeed at this." If medical professionals *do* happen to mention dietary changes, there is often little guidance or follow-up.

The thing is, I should have known better. At least this is what I sometimes tell myself. But the fact is, how could I have known? I was not taught, and the mixed messaging led me off course just like it does most of us. The people running my appointments were in the same boat I was in. They receive the same mixed messaging. Looking back, I wonder did I really need a nutritionist to tell me that carrots are better than Doritos? Why in the world are chips *ever* in my grocery cart even if as an "occasional" treat? Luckily, *now* I do know about practical, real ways to prevent and treat disease. These lifestyle modifications are what I want to share with you so that you can transform your health. What we eat and drink cause many of the top causes of death. We are not helpless victims of the aging process. We can choose food that nurtures our body.

One reason I sometimes think I should have known better is that I grew up in a big family and every summer we tended to a huge garden in our backyard. Not only did we eat fresh vegetables from the garden all summer, but we also froze and canned foods to be used through the winter. The main reason I got away from gardening was the misconception (or the party line conditioning) I had that it takes a lot of space. Now I grow lots of different vegetables in pots on my patio and a small, raised garden. Beets, kale, sweet potatoes, tomatoes, and peppers can all be potted plants.

Another reason I drifted from gardening was feeling that it was time consuming. It does take time – there is not a work around for that. When warm months come, I know that I will need to account for 30 minutes to an hour in my days to plant, water, weed, and harvest. Some days I will need more time than others. Gardening does take time and space, but not so much that I cannot grow at least *some* of my food.

I do not mean that everyone should grow their own garden. My point is, I know what real food looks like. I grew up knowing what the work looks like that goes into growing food. I suspect many people reading this book have the same experience, whether you have grown vegetables yourself or watched someone else do it. Yet somehow, as a society we have managed to get off track eating processed junk food. As a society, in agriculture, we have gotten off track focusing on quantity using monocropping, heavy fertilizers and pesticides, and bioengineering. In the end, we produce more than we use and much of it goes to waste.

FOOD LITMUS TEST

The test contains just two questions:

1. Does this food come from a plant?
2. Is it minimally processed?

If the answer to those two questions is yes, then it is real food. If not, simply turn up your nose, and keep walking.

Given how I was raised, how did I get so far away from eating whole plant foods?

Looking back, I realize that as an adult, I had picked up the notion that fruits and vegetables were expensive and hard to keep fresh. I do not think this was all my idea. I believe this is in the hidden messaging we hear over and over from the news media and the food industry. So gradually my grocery cart had less produce in it and more processed foods. I would buy things like fruit snacks, processed meat trays, cheese crackers, string cheese, yogurt, and fat filled, sugary granola bars for myself and my kids to take in our lunches. I worked nights and often I would grab crackers, microwave popcorn, or pretzels from a vending machine. Gradually, the more of these kinds of convenience snack foods that I bought, the less whole fruits and vegetables my family ate. The crazy part is, - I did not think we were eating bad. It crept up on me. Now, it is so obvious, but when it was happening, I thought since we were not eating fast-food for dinner every night that we were doing okay.

Speaking of fast-food, that is another thing that snuck up on me. Here is the thing, - we may not have been eating it for dinner, but we certainly were hitting the drive thru lines for a quick bite 4 or 5 days a week. As my kids had more activities on the calendar, we spent more time away from home and it started to become convenient to grab a $5 pizza, chicken dinners, or fast-food items off the dollar menu. This was like an "appetizer" to hold us over until we got home for a real meal. While, in my mind, I did not think we ate out often, the reality was that, at times, I was not cooking meals half of the days. It was not until I made the decision to eat less fast-food that I was faced with how many meals we were eating out. This also led me to reconsider whether fast-food was even a time saver. The lines can be long. Eating at a sit-down restaurant obviously can be time consuming too – wait for the server take your order, wait for the food to be prepared, wait for the server to bring the check, and wait for the server to process the payment.

When I did cook at home, we would have a salad, a starch, a meat, and a vegetable. So, at best we would have 2-3 servings of plant foods (not counting frozen French fries) 4 days a week and the rest of the days only 0-2 servings. That is a far cry from the low recommendations of 5-7 servings daily. When I looked around it seemed like we ate at home more than other families, so, you know, I was not comparing our nutrition to what healthy eating is, instead I was comparing our family to people who were eating even less healthy than we were. That is what gave me a false sense that we were eating healthy.

But it gets worse!

When I thought of making sure our family was eating nutritious food, I focused on eating protein. Except for peanut butter, I relied on meat, eggs, and dairy as protein sources. Now I know that it is more likely that we were eating *too much* protein than not enough. Yes, that is really a thing. The fact that there are health risks associated with too much protein is rarely mentioned in our American culture or by our experts at the Center of Disease Control and National Institute of Health. Even though these organizations are funded by taxpayer dollars, we are bombarded with messages about the importance of protein without more than a whisper of caution from them to say otherwise.

We are encouraged to eat meat and dairy, both of which are subsidized by taxpayers through our government. That presents a conflict of interest on many levels. I was surprised to learn when originally presented, the My Plate that is now recommended did not have meat or dairy on it. I have spent most of my life trusting these health organizations were watching out for my best interest. Unfortunately, now I feel my trust was misplaced as I discover how they allow their messages to be distorted by corporations and industry.

There is no mention in the mainstream culture of the fact too much protein can be harmful, and that animal protein is worse – even more so when cooked at high temperatures. Instead, to help support our animal-based protein consumption, there is the circulating myth that vegans and vegetarians do not get enough protein and are less healthy than those who eat animal products. What goes through your mind when you hear the word vegan or vegetarian? At this point, I cannot help but to believe any of the negative thoughts commonly associated with those words are the intentional result of purposeful conditioning by the meat industry. Studies have shown that plants do, in fact, provide enough protein for our bodies to function properly. Elephants, horses, gorillas, hippos, cows, deer, etc. – All grow and thrive on protein found in plants. Surely humans can too. Common plant foods contain 6-45% of calories as protein. The protein, carbohydrates, fiber, and fat found in plants are easily provided, at the levels our body needs, in a variety of plant foods.

When you look closer at restaurant menus for plant-based foods it is even more apparent how the myth of "more protein is better" surrounds us. I believe this "more protein" message is an important pillar in society because it helps support the need for the cruelty inflicted on animals raised for meat. By promoting protein and portraying animal rights activists in a negative light, industry manages to deflect responsibility for the poor conditions farm animals are raised in. This cruelty is presented as a necessary means to provide protein. *Another surprise for me was learn that the American Dietetic Association has said that it is **unnecessary** for humans to eat animal foods of any kind, at any stage, in our life.* We can get all the protein we need from plants. Hello? I do not believe that message has been broadcast adequately in the echo chambers… - Hello? Hello? Hello?

The convenient availability to eat out is not out there to support plant-based eaters. You can eat out and eat plant-based, but it takes the decision and mindfulness about what you are choosing to eat. I have found that the most nutritious meals are the ones made in my own kitchen, and nutritious food is what my body needs to function at its best. Though cooking at home does no always seem convenient, it can be, once you make the decision to do it.

Most people spend a lot of their time distracted which makes it easy to get off track and grab whatever is easiest. With intention, we can train our brains to pay more attention and be aware of what we are eating. When we bring this awareness to our food, we discover it is just as difficult to continue living unhealthily as it is to live healthy. We can pay attention and can make healthy convenient and fast. We can have both healthy and delicious food.

Knowing where we are beginning is essential for making decisions and creating our plan of action to get us to where we want to go. Considering our health before we hear words of caution from our doctor is easier than treating an established disease process. Also, we do not have to wait for our doctor to be concerned. We can be proactive in order that we do not reach the point of needing medications. Prevention before any signs or symptoms is ideal.

Whenever I begin working with a client, I start by finding out about their medical history and what is important to them. Take a minute and consider what you would like to change about your health. You can "choose your own adventure" and take a minute to read and consider how lifestyle impacts these specific areas now or keep reading and you will get to this information later in the book. These are diseases that can be treated and prevented with lifestyle.

Bowel Disease (Go to page 116)
Fatigue (Go to page 117)
Cancer (Go to page 118)
Alzheimer's (Go to page 119)

Liver Disease (Go to page 120)
Kidney Disease (Go to page 121)
Polycystic Ovary Disease (Go to page 122)
Diabetes or Borderline Diabetes (Go to page 123)
Chronic Inflammation/Autoimmune/Pain (Go to page 125)
Overweight (Go to page 126)
High Blood Pressure (Go to page 127)
Heart Disease (Go to page 127)

When was the last time you had your numbers checked?
It is okay if you do not know your numbers. Consider instead, how do you feel?

Are you sleeping well?

Do you have enough energy to get through the day? Do you have chronic fatigue?

Allergies? Sinusitis? Frequent colds? Frequent constipation or diarrhea? Headaches?

We do not have to focus on what our numbers are if we are focusing on feeling better. Numbers are helpful in gauging our progress and verifying that our actions are effective. Either approach will lead to healthy living if we take the following steps.

Instead of relying on medication to treat disease, we can prevent and treat much of America's disease and other illnesses with five lifestyle choices:

1. Eat a whole food plant-based diet - low in sugar, salt, and fat.
2. Be Active
3. Nurture our mind & relationships
4. Get proper rest
5. Eliminate alcohol, smoking, and drugs.

For now, if you are thinking *I don't want to do that* or *I don't think I can do all that*, - **Relax.**

Think of it this way. You already do these things. The goal is simply to increase the percentage of time you do them.

Your mind is one of your most powerful tools to achieving health. Do not let your mind sabotage your progress. Stop the limiting beliefs from playing in your head on a loop. As they say, "If you argue for your limits you get to keep them."

THOUGHT LITMUS TEST

The test contains just two questions:

1. Is it true?
2. Is continuing to think about this moving me forward in a positive manner?

If the answer to either of those two questions is no, then stop dwelling on it. Picture yourself in a sailboat and sail away to think about something else.

What we have done in the past is behind us. That was then. Our future does not depend on that. We determine our future by what we do now. We can start by continuing to create our plan for a healthy life. This is now.

We do not have to worry about our backstory in order to change our future. Too often we get stuck in our story forgetting we are the author. What we do today determines our health now and in the future.

So where are you at right now?

Date

_____

Height

_____

Weight

_____

BMI

_____

Blood Pressure

_____

Total Cholesterol

_____

HDL

_____

LDL

_____

Triglycerides

_____

Knowing where we start sets us up for positive reinforcement down the road. If we can see our numbers improving, it will help motivate us to continue on our path.

In the same way, if we *feel* better, we are motivated to remain dedicated to our decisions to live a healthy lifestyle. We can start making positive statements about it that begin positive feedback loops.

How do you feel?

Rate yourself by circling any of these that apply to you:

Fatigued? Poor sleep? Chronic constipation? Pain? Allergies? Frequent colds?

Is there anything you would like to improve? Headaches? Irritability?

What area do you most want to improve?

Has anything you tried worked for you in the past?

What are you currently doing to improve it?

How do you want to spend the rest of your life? Taking multiple medications to band-aid the problem?

Or would you rather prevent & fix problems at their root?

You can improve your health if you are brave enough to add a little adventure and get out of your comfort zone. You will find what you seek.

Carbs satisfy us:
Baked potato with salsa
No butter or sour cream

Read the next three lines out loud.
Read and repeat, as often as necessary.

I am taking care of my health today.

Write it down on a piece of paper and place it someplace you
will see it often. Each day is a gift we can use to begin again,
stretch to the next level, and be grateful for all that sparkles.

You are worth it!

CHAPTER THREE

Build An A-Team

*You reflect me in
Our daily conversations
And I reflect you*

Even if you feel you are healthy, staying healthy is a quest that never ends. Is it not?

Every adventure requires a team. Have you ever made a New Year's resolution to get in shape or lose fifteen pounds, set out with zest, only to lose momentum within 3 days? Our success can be interrupted by outside forces as we previously discussed. Other times we sabotage ourselves with our thought patterns and what we verbalize and choose to do.

To win the race with our plan, we need a team. Before we move forward it is helpful to acknowledge those people in our circle who are supportive of us. In addition, we need to identify people who have already been where we want to go. These will be people we can rely on as we move forward in part 2 to work on techniques to create healthy habits.

I once heard a keynote speaker at a graduation ceremony telling the new graduates to recognize the A-Team in their life.

71

Now when I think of the people in my life who love me day after day and always show up for me, I think of them as my A-Team. There is temptation to bask in our accomplishments as if we are solely responsible for them. The truth is, we all receive support in one way or another from people around us who are listening to us and supporting us. Not to mention the hand general providence can play as well.

One of my early memories is when I was around four years old. My younger brother was just born and home from the hospital and I was just getting to know him. One day, he woke up from sleeping and began to fuss. Before long the fussing escalated into the full blown strong and pitiful whole body crying that only an infant can manage. I began to cry too and called to my mom who was busy in the kitchen. She was probably irritated that now she had two babies crying. She poked her head into the room just long enough to tell me not to just stand there, but to talk to him and pat him. As I did, he was consoled and quieted as he listened to me tell him I was there and felt my little hand on him. I started to feel better too.

We do not need to be everything to everybody. The load is not that heavy. Obviously, my baby brother needed more that I could provide. We just need to recognize that our interactions with others impacts not just them, but also the people they interact with.

Sometimes that is all people need, - an ear to tell their story to. Someone who can share their experience and hardship. We are social creatures. We are all loved, all worthy, and we all make up the whole of humanity. When we know what brings meaning to our life in a world that sometimes seems all to meaningless, we build our mental resilience. We find our tribe, or A-team, and together we can overcome the challenges that face us.

We listen to others, and we also need to listen to our own God given wisdom and what our heart is calling us toward.

That is the voice to listen to! Think about the people you are having conversations with. Then find people who want the same things for you, and they will reinforce that voice. Have you heard the expression that it takes a village to raise a child? Think of that when you choose the people around you. People who have been where we want to go can help us get there. They are the village helping to raise you. We can make a difference for the people around us in return.

It makes a positive impact on our progress when those beside us "know the song in our heart and can sing it back to us when we have forgotten the words" (I think I have seen that embroidered on a pillow or apron somewhere). We want the people we choose to spend time with to act as a feedback loop to tell us whether we are putting in the actions needed to meet our goals. In other words, they help keep us honest with ourselves. The things we want in life do not magically happen – It takes effort, training, guidance, and commitment.

Have you ever had people say, "Oh, you are so lucky.." and you think, *no dude. This took a lot of blood, sweat, and tears.* Luck, blessing, and circumstance can play a role, but the work we put into achieving a goal is not irrelevant. Part of the work is when we invest in ourselves to build a team and new skills that help take us to the next level.

Due to each of us being born into our own unique set of circumstances, we are all running our own race. When we support each other through the good and the bad – that is when the magic happens. We want to surround ourselves with those who help us grow, not those who are trying to control us. If we are in a place where we are not looking to grow, we cannot really be helped because we do not even know we need help. I am going to assume that most readers of this book do not fall into this category. More likely, most of us fall into the category of knowing we have a problem and knowing we need help, but sometimes we do not fully understand what questions to ask, or we lack motivation and support to make changes.

Therefore, a good team that includes people we want to try to be like is important. We also need people who can help us help ourselves. These are the people who can act best as mentors. They have already formed the habit of doing something that other people without their success do not like to do. They serve as role models by modeling the behaviors we want to add to our life to reach our goals. Making a habit of their winning behaviors can help propel us to where they are.

What are they doing that you are not doing? Instead of being jealous or envying what they have, we can copy it.

What do you appreciate most about your family and friends?

Who is on the same journey that you are on and how can you better connect with them?

Who can you count on to care, listen, support, encourage, love, and accept you?

Think about how you are making a difference in the lives of others. Our energy can pick others up in the same way that they make us feel good. Just by spending time together and getting to know each other we nurture our relationships. Then these healthy connections with others make our lives happier. Studies have shown laughter is able to reduce pain, reduce blood pressure, and increase our energy. Be the person who lightens the lives of those around you. Pick people for your team who you are comfortable sharing your thoughts with. As you spend time together, you each understand where the other is coming from. Taking time to look at things from another's point of view helps us discover solutions and processes that work best.

Maybe you are at a point of isolation in your life. The last couple of years has left many people feeling alone. We may feel alone at times, but every day we have the opportunity to see ourselves in others. See their struggles, see their dreams, and see their beauty. We can help them with their sadness, give them a hand up, and help *them* find new adventure. Trust yourself and choose to reflect love next time you find yourself sitting next to someone different. Being brave enough to initiate a conversation could be the beginning of a connection that lasts only a moment, or one that lasts for years.

These lasting relationships require establishing and maintaining trust. It takes time to build trust. We have to show that we will do what we say we are going to do and our actions reflect the values that we proclaim to value. This goes not just for our relationships with others, but also our relationship with ourselves. Once we have trust we do not want to break it. Although trust can be repaired, broken trust takes more time to heal. To keep our relationships strong, we must avoid actions that can cause distrust in others like lying, omitting information, or not doing what we have previously agreed to do.

Transparency is a word that gets thrown around an awful lot lately. I am afraid it might be beginning to lose its meaning. I believe transparency goes along with setting expectations. Unless you say it, others may not know what your expectations are. After you have known someone and spent time building trust for at least 4 to 6 months you may find yourselves developing a common language – those heart songs - and can even do some mind-reading.

If you want to grow your circle with these meaningful relationships, you may need to put yourself out there and be vulnerable. Volunteer for a cause you believe in. Take a yoga class or join a club. Exploring new hobbies is a sure way to have the opportunity to smile, say hello, introduce ourselves and start a new relationship. Invite someone to get together.

The way to meet and get to know people is to make the decision to do it. Look at upcoming area events and sign up to participate in a 5K walk, color run, paddle fest, fat tire or other activity you would enjoy or do something else in your community. Go to the library. Participate in a clean-up day. Sign up for a class or education day on some interest you have. Look at upcoming community events. Think virtually. Sometimes mentors can be those you have never even met or talked to, but if their story inspires you, follow it from afar. Even if you do not come away with lasting friends you can benefit from being surrounded by others who you share some values with. Signing up puts a date on the calendar and makes you more likely to get moving to prepare.

Is there anyone who I blame, nag, badger, punish, coerce, manipulate, or criticize to get what I want?

Or am I simply stuck in inaction?

What changes can I make to let those behaviors go?

Whose A-team am I on? Who is on my A-team?

These two teams have overlap. There are most likely people we show up for who are not really there for us, but we know it is important to us to be there for them.

A bowl of oatmeal,
Microwave with water, add fruit
-Like blueberries - Yum!

Take a moment to sit still. Pay attention to your breath.
Pay attention to how your body feels.
Do not judge it, just feel it.

Read the next line out loud.
The words you speak shape the life in front of you.

Read and repeat, as often as necessary.

I am grounded in love.

I am grateful for the people in my life.

CHAPTER FOUR

Follow Your Path

Get what you ask for.
Develop awareness of
the dream you pursue.

Now that you have your team together where is it that you are going?

Where do you want to go?

What do you need to get there?

Have you asked for it and trust it will be provided to you? (God is polite and does not barge into our lives. He waits for us to ask him to come into it.)
Have you ever felt like you spend more time watching other people having grand adventures than having your own? We want flavor in our life the same way we want flavor in our food. Planning for activity in our life gives us clarity we need to follow our own path of adventure.

I have noticed that in some ways people tend to lose themselves as they age. It starts in high school when we start feeling the pressure to pick a career path. Once we are on that path it becomes a big part of our identity. There is nothing wrong with that. Especially if your career path is something that fills you up. If we get married and have children, we can lose ourselves even more. Instead of pursuing our own hobbies and dreams, we nurture our children to grow through a variety of activities and become more heavily invested in theirs rather than our own. We end up over identifying with our duty role and responsibilities rather than attending to our own needs. The chaos and noise in the world can make us forget who we are.

I always say the day of my daughter's accident was a turning point for me to lifestyle medicine. But the signposts had been on my journey all along. Several years prior to her accident I participated in a mothers of preschoolers group. One day we had a speaker come in who talked about taking time to develop our hobbies. Really? I had four kids, two under five. My main hobby was laundry. We did some group activities where we remembered our childhood and what we liked to do. Sing, run, paint, read, sew, hike, swim, write, - I discovered I had all sorts of potential hobbies, but I was not allowing time for them. I have dabbled off and on in art and writing over the years. That day I became more aware of putting activities I enjoy back into my life. I began doing simple things. Instead of watching ball practice, I would take a walk while my son's team practiced. I began carrying a book with me to have handy for times in my day that I was stuck waiting.

Remember who you are.

When I started my lifestyle-is-medicine journey I was already on board with the idea of increasing activity in my life and I began putting more activities I enjoy back into my schedule. I walk daily, and in recent years have done significantly more hiking, swimming, running, writing, and reading. Those are just some of the things I enjoy. Think about what you would like to do more of. Do you play a musical instrument? Do you enjoy drawing, puzzles, walking the dog, crosswords, or birding? What gives you a thrill inside? What activities do you get lost in?

One of my patients shared with me that when she gave up smoking cigarettes she continued to go outside and sit as she always had to smoke. Instead of smoking, she told me how she sat on the bench in her backyard and fed the birds and squirrels. That led her to other interests because her backyard was near an old canal. She then started researching and walking parts of the old canal system in her state and she made new friends in the process.

It is never too late to develop a hobby or dig deeper into what interests you. Another patient of mine was in her eighties and while talking with her I discovered she was an expert on Mesopotamia. She revealed she had not always been. It was only in the last 10 years of her life that she began to learn, teach, and speak about the history of Mesopotamia. She noted that Mesopotamia is such a niche topic that it was not hard to become well-known because only a small circle of interested people are involved. Pursuing her interest helped keep her engaged, moving, and active.

When thinking of adding activity to your life, try not to associate activity with weight or weight loss. Activity is what we get to do after we fuel our body with nutritious food. Part of the hidden narrative we receive from multiple media sources is that if we just move more, we will lose weight and be healthy. While it is true that building muscle helps us to burn calories, you will have a much greater impact on maintaining a healthy weight by eating low calorie, nutritious food. It takes an awful lot of jogging to burn one pound of fat.

In your mind, unlink exercise and weight. Instead, associate food with weight. Then couple food with fuel for exercise too.

Anti-inflammatories provided in plants helps to cut workout recovery times. Plant-based foods are less fat, which improves blood flow and provides athletes with increased endurance through better oxygenation of muscles. Carbohydrates found in plants provide glucose that can be stored for energy as glycogen. That is the reason athletes load with carbs like pasta, bread, rice, or sweet potatoes a day or two before an event.

People think "carbs make you fat." How many times a day do we hear that message? Despite the story we have been told, carbohydrates do not make us fat. The truth is, some of the extra carbs that are taken in are stored as glycogen and the rest are eliminated as heat. On the other hand, extra fat taken in is stored as fat on our body. It may seem like carbohydrates are the problem because they are usually eaten with fat. Take the butter, cheese, and sour cream off the baked potato and top instead with oil free salsa, mustard, or nutritional yeast. The carbohydrates get burned and there is no excess fat to store. Fat (think added oils) makes us fat.

Food helps to maintain a healthy weight, and food helps to fuel our body so we can do the activities and work we enjoy. If you do not know what you enjoy, that is okay. Being a beginner is hard. It can be confusing and stressful whether we are learning a sport, learning to build, learning an instrument, or learning to make different lifestyle choices. If it seems like it is going to take a lot of know-how, start small. Sometimes we do not even know what questions to ask. Being a beginner requires setting our ego aside. It requires some determination and patience.

And mental toughness! People talk about eating a whole elephant as a strategy for developing mental toughness. The idea is not to focus on eating the elephant in its entirety. Just focus on the next bite. Or as others might say, just do the next right thing.

Though it has its difficulties, at the same time, being a beginner is easy because you do not have to have all the answers. Mistakes are expected. I find myself starting as a beginner over and over as I get older, not just in hobbies, but in work too. Allowing yourself to be a beginner or explore new areas can be fun. You do not have to be good at everything to enjoy it or learn from it. Just because you start something does not mean you have to finish it or do it forever. Just the willingness to go there may lead to new connections, conversations, and opportunities that you have not yet imagined.

Being open to growth and having a willingness to learn is what gets us through the beginner phase. You do not have to have all the answers. Ask for help and if you mess up – try again. Be kind to yourself. Looking foolish is often a fear, but everyone stinks in the beginning. Allowing yourself to be a beginner is allowing yourself to leave fear behind and be brave. Being a beginner is a new start! It is an opportunity for growth by observing, asking questions, making mistakes, and moving forward.

As you consider activities or work you might like or have enjoyed in the past, recognize that it is okay not to be perfect at it. I am wrong about things every day and it is okay. Whenever we try new things there is a learning curve. We just have to be humble enough to admit it, learn from it, and plan to do better the next time. Think about it. If someone you know makes a mistake and must start over or redo a project, do you think they are a total failure? Probably not. Especially not if it is new to them. Golf, tennis, running, knitting, flying a helicopter, woodworking, bowling - whatever it is – any time we take up a new activity, we have to give ourselves time to get through the learning curve.

Sometimes good enough is good enough. We cannot sweat *every*thing or we will not have time and energy to sweat the most important things.

Even with all the changes I have made in my life, I still sometimes find myself burdened with the pressure to "find purpose." For me, it is easier to find what excites me and then start doing it. Maybe if it benefits me, I can find a way to help it benefit others in the future. When we find a way to make the grind fun, the work can be the reward. We become committed to the journey more than the destination or goal. The MOPS group speaker also talked about how when we are younger, we do not think so hard about what we enjoy and like to do. It is only as we grow older, approaching graduation and the beginning of our work career that we feel the pressure to chase one thing. The truth is, we all wear more than one hat. We can choose to do more than one thing. We each have unique gifts that bring joy into our lives and the lives of others.

Purpose does not have to be scary. When we take time to see the purpose of smaller activities in our lives it helps us to become grounded in a larger purpose. When you are doing simple activities that you repeat day after day or week to week ask yourself why. Why are you taking out the trash? Why are you doing the dishes? Why do you cut the grass? Why do you go to work? As you drill down (like a toddler) why? Why? Why? You become more aware of what you are doing and what motivates you to do it.

It is not enough to know what we want. We need to believe we are worthy of receiving it. Work can be recreation. Just as recreation can be work. Different activities bring different reactions to each of us. You do not have to pick based on what others pick. There is room to be the same and there is room for differences. We all make mistakes. We all fall short, but we are all valuable. Recognize and do the work required to get where you want to go. Every one of us is a part of one magnificent world. We are each equally deserving of receiving what we ask and work for.

Keep in mind, when it comes to activity in our lives, I am not necessarily talking about a rigorous exercise program or learning something new. Being active means doing something you enjoy that involves movement. If it has aerobic benefits, then all the better. Being active can go a long way to improving your state of mind which will only help you on your journey to better health.

Our body is closely connected with our identity and how we think of ourselves. Though what we can do with our body impacts our thoughts about ourselves, we are more than our body. If we lose a body part, get injured, lose or gain weight, or even simply get a dramatic new haircut, we are still the same person. It helps me sometimes to step back and think about what adventures I value beyond the physical aspects of them.

To find clarity for your adventures write down some activities you currently enjoy, used to enjoy, or have always wanted to try. Rather than thinking of exercise as work, think of what you enjoy that involves moving your body – bicycling, walking, running, kayaking, hiking, basketball, soccer, jogging – what is your game? What do you enjoy that brings you mental energy?

_____

_____

_____

Recognize what is getting in the way. Addictions from chapter 1?

_____

_____

_____

Saboteurs? Ourselves. If it is others who are stopping us, we can find mentors who will support us elsewhere. If we want to make room for activity we enjoy in our lives, we must want it more than we want those things. Then we must make the decision to create a plan to do what it takes to get it and begin speaking about it.

I want _____ more than I want _____ and I trust myself to take action to get _____ by doing these things _____.

Visualize what you want your daily activity to be.

Imagine what family and friends you want to share your time with.

What kind of work fills you up? What activities do you enjoy? When do you feel like you are in your groove?

Back to chapter one again. How is it that you start your day? Is there room to add an activity that will bring more health and satisfaction into your life?

Tomorrow your morning can look different. Consider writing in a new line.

First, I eat a bowl of oatmeal.

Then I get dressed.

Then I go for a 10-minute walk outside. If it is raining, I will stretch inside.

Then I _____.

Dinner made easy
Slice and sauté peppers, Add
Rice, spice, and red beans

Read the next line out loud. Repeat throughout your day, as often as necessary. The spoken word has an impact on your actions.

I release the struggle.

I am grateful for my body, my mind, and nutritious food that fuels my day.

Think about it and take it out into the world and live it. Turn it into a new frontier in your life.

CHAPTER FIVE

Lighten Your Load

I know where I am
I have a plan and intend
To act on it now

So far, we have assessed our current health and considered where we want to go with it and what activities we want our health to allow us to participate in. We have considered the power of mindset. We have identified our A-team. Now is the time to create the goals that will help us achieve our vision.

So often in American medicine we elevate doctors and medical professionals. The goals they set for us become our goals. This elevation will sometimes make even our A-team discourage us from attempting to manage our health independently. When others try to criticize, it is important to be true to yourself and do what you can for your health. You are responsible for activities you choose to participate in every day. You are responsible for what you drink. You are responsible for what goes into your mouth. You are responsible for creating a space where you can relax and thrive. You are responsible for keeping your space clean. Trust yourself to take care of yourself. When you are grounded in your vision and purpose you do not need to be afraid of what others will think.

A good plan helps lighten our load.

I believe we each need to have a more active role in setting goals for our health. If you do not know what you want, you cannot get there. We need to put ourselves on the same level with our medical professionals. They have a role to play in our health, but it does not overshadow our own role! Traditionally, when I work with clients, I guide them to use SMART goals. Maybe you have heard of this method. Another method with a similar concept is WOOP goals.

The letters in WOOP stand for **w**ish, **o**utcome, **o**bstacle, **p**lan. When using WOOP, first, set time aside to think of what would be the best **wish** that could happen to you over the next four weeks. Then summarize it in 4 to 6 words. It does not have to be a four-week timeframe depending on what your wish is. Pick a timeframe that is appropriate. Sometimes bigger wishes with longer timeframes can be broken into smaller wishes.

Next, consider how you will feel or how your life will be different because of that wish coming true. In other words, what is the **outcome** of the wish? Summarize it in 4 to 6 words. Being able to summarize the outcome of a wish shows how much you care about a wish. If you are not able to imagine the outcome, consider if the wish is more important for other people in your life than yourself.

Now consider what stands between you and your wish. Are there any behaviors or inner **obstacles** you can change that will help you achieve the wish? Summarize obstacles into 4 to 6 words. Lastly, think of a thought or action you can take to overcome the obstacles. Phrase it in an if-then **plan** statement. For example, **if** the meeting runs late and I do not have time to take a walk after work, **then** I will take one after dinner. **If** I go to eat at the Italian restaurant, **then** I will eat spaghetti with meatless sauce and a salad. **If** I want to eat dessert, **then** I will eat a piece of fruit. **If** I find myself mindlessly scrolling through tv channels, **then** I will turn off the tv and take a walk or do any meal prep for tomorrow. If-then statements help us with big obstacles as well as small ones. We can add them as we encounter obstacles we have not thought of.

My favorite part of WOOP goals are the if-then statements. They also work well when creating a plan for **SMART** goals. The letters in SMART stand for **S**pecific, **M**easurable, **A**chievable, **R**elevant, **T**imely. For instance, I could say, "Patient's goal is to improve their A1C," but 1 to 3 months down the road how will I know if they have met the goal? A SMART goal would be, "Patient's goal is to have 3 A1C levels less than 7% in the next 9 months."

A SMART goal states specifically what we want to happen and when we want it to happen. Whether the goal is achievable or reasonable is decided by experience. Someone who currently walks 20 minutes a day will have different activity goals than someone who cannot walk 5 minutes without becoming short of breath and fatigued. Obviously different people have different barriers as well. Considering barriers helps to evaluate whether a goal is achievable. Sometimes barriers are known and sometimes you may discover them along the way. It is okay if barriers are not all identified initially. Just do your best to identify anticipated barriers. In part two we will address common barriers I have seen in my work: decreased motivation, knowledge deficit, travel, family/friends, time, and money. Barriers are important to identify accurately because they are what we need to overcome to meet our goals.

Other barriers are not as easy to validate. Am I not meeting this goal because I am not motivated or, do I simply need more information? Am I not meeting this goal because I do not have the funds, or do I have money that I am spending elsewhere that I could put toward this goal? Am I not meeting this goal because I do not have the knowledge of what needs to be done, or is it that there is something out of my control that is stopping me? The fact is not all barriers are within our control. Barriers do not have to be within our control but identifying what is and is not within our power to change is important when creating an action plan or interventions for our goals. Ideally, we want to create goals that we have power over.

For instance, I might say I want to get my book published by the end of 2022. However, this depends on other people. Both what the publisher is looking for and who else is submitting their manuscript at the same time is out of my control. I can take steps to research publishers and what they are looking for, but that does not eliminate my competition. A better goal might be to say I will research twenty-five publishers and submit my manuscript to the 5 that are most appropriate within the next 2 months. Or I could start with the original goal and as I am creating an action plan, I would then address those areas that I can control.

Identifying barriers such as decreased motivation, fear, and lack of confidence fall into this category. Identifying these barriers takes honest self-evaluation and can be addressed and overcome just as any other barrier can. It is important to realize when mindset barriers are present so that you can include interventions in your action plan to retrain your brain to approach your goal with a constructive mindset and resilience.

Resilience is important because we need to recognize and reinforce our ability to bounce back. Struggle is a part of life, and we need compassion – from ourselves and from each other. Our resilience reflects our ability to accept the good in life and hunt the good stuff when necessary. Joy and grief can exist simultaneously in life. Being resilient allows us to block grief and loss from ruining what is good in our lives. Sometimes we are not even the one directly impacted, and we still feel suffering and loss for others. When we know ourselves and act deliberately, we build our ability to act and think flexibly to overcome our barriers.

There are different reasons to get distracted or drawn off track. Five of the biggies are:

- Family
- Cost
- Time
- Availability
- Know How

If time and money were not an issue, what would I do?

_____

_____

_____

Who is preventing me from improving my health? How can I talk to them about it?

_____

_____

_____

It does not really matter which method of goal setting you decide to use if you are taking the time to set measurable goals to build a plan around. I usually set long and short goals. Think of it as what you can do right now, this year, and someday. Take time to write them down. Written goals are more likely to be acted on.

Block time for planning. Fridays are a good day to plan for the upcoming week and focus on next items to be completed for short term goals that lead to meeting long term goals.

Block time for evaluating. Mondays are a good day to reflect on the past week.

Resting is important. Plan time for rest and relaxation. Use your purpose as your foundation and each small action fuels your productivity to supporting your purpose. When we give ourselves rest it helps us stay connected to the big picture of our life and keeps us from getting weary by peaks and valleys of our life because we have a clear picture of where we are going. When we expect ups and downs, we can plan to give ourselves time for the rest we need to stay the course.

A can of lentils
Pepper and onion, saute,
Add tomato sauce

Read the next line out loud. Repeat throughout your day, as often as necessary. The spoken word has an impact on your actions.

I ignite my creativity.

I choose the path that I follow.

Not another chapter!

Before we go any further, how about we uncover and debunk the hidden messages and myths we may have rolling around in our brains?

As I made the lifestyle changes that jumpstarted my own health, I had to tackle some common myths or hidden messages that I had been operating under. I have no doubt you are operating under at least a few of these too. These myths can be intentional, promoted by some groups or businesses for their benefit, and then unintentionally parroted by culture, policy, and systems as a result. Other myths may be unintentional, but direct our culture, systems, and actions just the same.

Before my daughter's accident I had accepted that declining health was part of getting older. That was the first myth I busted. (Again: Please note that if you are taking medications, it is best to work with your doctor when introducing lifestyle changes as they may need to adjust your doses as your health improves.)

Myth #1 "Declining health is part of getting older."

Wrong. I had subscribed to this myth without thinking about it. It seems reasonable because I was witnessing declining health in myself, in my patients, and in those around me as we aged. But when I began researching lifestyle medicine,

I realized there were plenty of people who managed to age without increased disability in their retirement years. The Blue Zones of the world are the areas where people have the longest lifespans. Some researchers have taken time to pinpoint what these zones have in common that allow their communities to be healthier without the large number of people with chronic disease we see in most of America and other countries. They have been looking to learn what it is that makes these places the unexpected, successful exception to the failing norms of health in the rest of the world. Within the United States, the Adventists in Loma Linda community has been a source of study as their community is one of these Blue Zones. It turns out that the people living in Blue Zones commonly have four areas where they have similar approaches to life.

- place importance on belonging to both family and community
- eat with a plant slant avoiding meat and added sugars
- know your purpose, but know how to relax
- move naturally throughout the day.

Many of the chronic diseases we see in the United States are a result of lifestyle choices related to nutrition, exercise, and relationships. When I took control and adjusted my habits around these choices, I began to see a decrease in weight gain, high blood pressure, and insulin resistance. I improved my mobility, cognition, and risk for heart disease. Along with that, I have more energy and less of the aches and pains that I had previously come to accept as part of the aging process.

How would your life be different if you did not accept declining health as part of the aging process? Would it be worth it to consider nutrition, exercise, relationships, and mindfulness as methods to support better health in your life?

Deteriorating health as I age is not a "given."

Myth #2 "Everything in moderation for a balanced healthy life."

Wrong. This is another myth I had subscribed to big time. On the surface it sounds reasonable. When I began to put thought into it, I realized that of course there are some things that I do not need at all. Like alcohol for instance. I do not need beer, wine, or spirits in my life to survive. Also, I do not really need to watch television or scroll through social media at all. I do not need baked goods, or potato chips to survive. I do not need caffeine drinks or energy "shots" in moderation for health either. Also, I do not really need people or businesses in my life who are constantly trying to get me to do things that are not in my best interest.

The reality is that the notion of "everything in moderation" ignores the fact that some activities, foods, and people in our lives are toxic. Some things are bad habits. For example, non-alcoholic fatty liver disease (NAFLD) is now the most common chronic liver disease affecting 1 in 3 adults in the United States. It is associated with the consumption of soft drinks and meat. Some experts cite that even one soda a day can raise the odds of NAFLD by 45%. Not to offend the soda industry, but at those odds, does soda "in moderation" make sense? Not to mention, whose definition of moderation are we using? Does the same definition apply to each thing?

Recognizing that I have the choice to remove unhealthy foods and drinks from my life was a powerful step in being accountable for my health. I choose what activities I participate in, and I choose the people I spend my time with. I do not need toxicity just for the sake of balance.

My health changed for the better when I started paying more attention to the choices I was letting big businesses make for me. Although I used to enjoy the addictive foods and beverages that they promote, I do not think their products are worth risking my health for. When I give myself room to always have unhealthy products as a choice, I create frustration and negative emotions within me. Removing them from my life altogether rather than trying to consume them in moderation reduces the yo-yo back and forth having to try to have enough willpower to withstand cravings. Getting rid of them altogether makes it easier to deal with.

If I do end up eating something that I consider unhealthy I put it behind me and move on. Which is different than allowing myself to eat it more frequently but "in moderation."

Myth #3 "Milk does the body good."

Wrong. This myth has been ingrained in my head since kindergarten when they served us those cute little cartons of milk every morning and again in the afternoon at snack time. Reinforcement of the myth continued through grade school and into nursing school and into adulthood and parenthood. The truth is, cows get the calcium in their milk from the plants they eat, and I can get all the calcium that I need from eating plants too. The dairy industry relies on us believing that milk is the best source of calcium. This myth is reinforced by the dairy industry and our government simply because the industry is profitable and lobbies from the industry impact how policy is written.

Not only can I get the nutrients milk provides from elsewhere, but when I choose not to drink milk or eat dairy products, I am also not getting things that I do not need for my health that are found in dairy. Casein is a protein found in dairy milk that has been shown to promote cancer and has also been strongly linked to some autoimmune diseases. Casomorphins found in milk have proved to be addictive, making us crave dairy products, like cheese, for instance.

The high fat content in dairy products can lead to insulin resistance and other diseases such as high blood pressure, heart disease, fatty liver disease, increased body fat, weight gain, and other chronic conditions. Consuming dairy products also means taking in the cow's hormones which can have a negative effect on my body. Cow's milk also contains six times more insulin-like growth factor (a promoter of tumor growth) than human milk. If I choose to drink cow's milk, medications that have been given to the cow are also passed on to me, as well as pesticides, heavy metals, other toxins, and bacteria.

Now that I no longer consume dairy products regularly, my persistent sinus congestion has disappeared, and I can breathe easier. I had forgotten how it feels to be able to breathe in deeply through my nose! Many others find that their stomach pains and irregularities with their bowels improve.

We have a culture that portrays lactose intolerance as abnormal even though our bodies were not designed to drink milk or consume dairy for life. A human mother's milk is designed for the initial growth of our body in the first few years of our life. During this time our body produces the lactase enzyme to help digest lactose. As we grow out of the toddler years, our body begins to decline in its production of lactase. That is why about 75% of the global population is lactose intolerant. Being able to digest lactose is the exception. In short, humans were never meant to consume milk products after the natural age of weaning, and it does not do our body any extra good to do so.

Specifically, our bones have long been cited as reason to consume dairy, but there is some question to the truth of that assertion. A recent large analysis published in the British Medical Journal in 2015 concluded: "Dietary calcium intake is not associated with risk of fracture, and there is no clinical trial evidence that increasing calcium intake from dietary sources prevents fractures. Evidence that calcium supplements prevent fractures is weak and inconsistent." Allegedly, after Doctor Spock turned vegan at ninety-one years old, he revised his previous recommendations for dairy intake in his famous book: "Baby and Child Care", stating cows' milk should not be fed to infants and clarifying he no longer would recommend dairy products. He reasoned that other calcium sources offer many advantages that dairy products do not.

Rather than dairy or infant formula, most everyone agrees human breastmilk has the perfect balance of nutrients for infants. It is high in fat (about 35% of calories), low in protein (5%), and 60% carbs - mainly lactose (which remember, - we begin to lose our ability to digest after about 2 and a half years old). An infant will easily double its birthweight within 6 months on a breastmilk diet. Under the age of three, infants and children require more fat in their diets than adults.

Beyond macros, - breast milk also contains antibodies, prebiotics, enzymes, and glycoproteins. Not to mention it magically changes its composition over time to meet a baby's needs. The World Health Organization recommends breastfeeding until at least age 2, estimating this advice could significantly impact childhood mortality worldwide. If breastmilk is unavailable, most children over 1 year can get the nutrition they need from whole foods and water. Yet somehow our culture has moved away from breastfeeding and toward formula and cow's milk. This has not served us well, and not only that, it makes our families vulnerable when formula is found to be tainted and production suddenly ceases as we have seen happen in recent years.

Humans are the *only species on earth* drinking milk after weaning. We know lactose, casein, estrogen, progesterone, insulin-like growth factor, pesticides, heavy metals, and toxins found in dairy is not desirable. Yet, our status quo continues to promote the myth and recommends serving cow's milk up several times a day. One cup of 2% milk has 295 mg of calcium and one cup of whole milk has 276 mg. Plant-based foods provide far more calcium without the negative effects milk has.

Consider calcium in other common plant foods:
1 cup almond milk = 450mg
1 cup tofu = 516mg
1 cup cooked collard greens = 358mg
1 cup cooked spinach = 244mg.

Surprising, right? It is possible to bust the myth that milk does the body good and switch to a milk alternative. The hidden message that milk is the best food to provide calcium does not hold up. Oat, soy, and almond are alternative milks that are quickly becoming more available. Sometimes they come with stories that plant-based milks are bad for the environment, but the question is, compared to what? When compared with the environmental impacts of dairy product their impact is far less in land use, greenhouse gas emissions, freshwater use, and runoff into water system.

You may be surprised to learn that hip fractures are most common where meat consumption is most high. Meat increases acid load in the body whereas plants increase base load. The body must maintain a tight acid base balance. When we eat meat, bones become the primary buffer to neutralize acid in the body. Osteoporosis can be one of the end results of dissolving bones to protect our acid base balance. At the same time calcium builds up in the urine leading to kidney stones. Meat consumption put together with lack of exercise and high caffeine intake, which are both common to Americans, leads to weak bones and more fractures.

I was taught from a young age by government agencies and the dairy industry that cow's milk should be a part of my diet. I was eating cheese, yogurt, butter, sour cream, drinking milk and thinking dairy was doing my body good. All the while the opposite was true. The fat, salt, and hormones helped lead to weight gain, high blood pressure, and food addiction. Only when I removed it did I see the truth in how unhealthy it is.

Milk *does not* do the body good. Dairy products can lead to food allergies, cancer, autoimmune disease, infectious disease, calcium loss, kidney stones, respiratory congestion, inflammation, and osteoporosis. If you take nothing else away from this book, take away the idea of cutting all dairy products from your life and put it into action! Then watch your body's health dramatically improve.

Myth #4 "Carbohydrates cause high blood sugar."

Wrong. Over 80 years ago doctors were aware that fat decreased insulin activity. Yet sugar gets the blame for diabetes. This myth continues to be spread by the current healthcare system. Fat in our diet, *not carbohydrates*, causes insulin resistance which can lead to type two diabetes. Fat we eat can build up in cells making it hard for sugar to move from our bloodstream into our cells. People think high sugar is the problem, but the problem is the fat buildup *preventing* the sugar from entering cells by blocking insulin. The fat is gumming up the lock that insulin uses to allow sugar in. Get rid of the fat, and the sugar can be used. High blood sugars are the result of fat in our blood and muscles.

For most of my nursing career, I was dead wrong on this. I was taught to teach diabetics to count and limit carbohydrates with not much distinction between simple carbohydrates and complex carbohydrates. The mindset was carbs are carbs. I even went as far as to recommend this to people in general as a healthy way to eat. I thought everyone would be healthier if they subscribed to a diabetic diet, limiting pastas, breads, baked goods, potatoes, rice, etc. Limiting refined carbohydrates found in pastries and the oils that come with them is good. However, there is no reason to limit potatoes, sweet potatoes, and whole grains. Lumping all carbohydrates together as equal is not helpful. Starch and fiber are good for health. All the powerful antioxidants fruits can provide are good for health. The vitamins and minerals in starchy vegetables are good for health. Fiber and starch fill us up and satisfy hunger.

Type two diabetes is caused by too much fat in the blood and muscles. This fat prevents insulin from doing its job of moving glucose from the blood into our cells. Diets high in processed foods and animal products contribute to increased fat in the body. (Also, animal protein has been shown to contribute to kidney disease and calcium loss.) The popular treatment of a high-fat, low-carbohydrate diet can cause insulin resistance. Which could be why we are seeing our incidence of diabetes going up, not down. It is not well publicized, but much research instead points to a low-fat, plant-based, whole-food diet which includes natural carbohydrates such as those in sweet potatoes, carrots, corn, and oats for good health.

Carbohydrates provide energy.

Myth #4 "Exercise is the best way to lose weight."

Wrong. This myth was one that took me the most time to come to terms with. When thinking of adding activity to my life, I had learned to associate activity with weight or weight loss. Now I think of exercise as activity I *get to do* after I fuel my body with nutritious food. Part of the controlled narrative or hidden message I continue to receive from multiple media sources is that if I just move more, I will lose weight and be healthy.

While it is true that building muscle helps to burn calories, I have a much greater impact on maintaining a healthy weight by eating low calorie nutritious food. It is food that causes weight gain. Too many calories lead to weight gain. Connect good nutrition with energy for exercise. When I eat higher quality food, I feel better, I move better, and the muscle I build helps with the afterburn effect.

The best way to lose weight is to eat low calorie plant-based nutrient dense foods. Fruits, vegetables, whole grains, potatoes, and legumes are full of the nutrients my body needs without the excess fat that it does not need. I eat nutritious food, and I use that as fuel for natural movement. Blue Zones incorporate natural movement in their day. Exercise such as walking, running, and lifting are as much a part of my daily routine as eating and sleeping.

Do not underestimate these natural movements as a form of exercise. This simple exercise can maintain strength and balance, boost our mood, and relieve mild depression or blues. If we are not busy maintaining, then we are going backwards – like standing still on a treadmill. To keep up, we must keep moving forward.

Myth #6 "Some oils are healthy."

Wrong. You might think, "*But I thought our body needed fat? And what about coconut oil, grapeseed oil, and olive oil? Aren't those healthy?*"

The list goes on of oils that have been presented in a positive light. However, all oils are processed making them calorie dense. Consider that plant-based foods, fruits to legumes, are less than 1,000 calories per pound. Oils, on the other hand, are 4,000 calories per pound! Any oil is nothing but fat. It has no water and no fiber. It contains nothing to fill you up. Less oil means less calories which equals less weight gain.

Research indicates that the human body is designed to eat 3 to 5 pounds of food a day totaling about 2,000 calories. I do not need to spend my day counting calories because I now simply understand that oils are super processed plant fragments that add excess calories quickly without adding nutrition. Avoid those added oils and most of the excess calorie problem is solved! The fats found in plants will meet my body's need for fat.

Most of the world lives on basic carbohydrate starch: corn, rice, beans, potatoes, oats, wheat, etc. which are somewhere around five hundred calories a pound. Fruits are about three hundred calories a pound. Vegetables are around two hundred calories a pound. Raw salads are about one hundred calories a pound. Without counting calories, just keep in mind that you will be able to consume the 3 to 5 pounds of food your body desires without exceeding the calories it needs. Simply avoid small weights of food that are high in calories because they contain oil.

I used to be like a moth to a flame, I was drawn to these high calorie foods because my brain, like yours, is wired to seek the most calories with the least amount of work. Let us face it. When we dump oil and butters into our meals, they taste better to us. However, I was not designed to consume oil any more than I was designed to consume soda pop.

When you hear people refer to studies that say olive oil (or whichever oil they are promoting) is healthier, think, *"Compared to what?"* If the studies are comparing olive oil to other oils and saturated fats, then yes, it may come out ahead because olive oil, for instance, is only 14 percent saturated fat. Chicken and beef fat are 30 and 50 percent saturated fat. However, if a study were to compare a diet filled with olive oil to one that omits oil, then it would be logical that the no-oil diet would win because it is lower in unnecessary calories and would not have the damaging impact on the lining of blood vessels which result from saturated fat. Therefore, it causes less weight gain, and less chronic disease such as heart disease and diabetes.

Now I recognize my body can get all the fats it needs in the right amount from eating a variety of whole plant-based foods.

Myth #7 "The more protein, the better."

Wrong. Extra protein taken in is eliminated through our kidneys. Overeating protein can hurt our kidneys. Excess animal protein is acid producing in our bodies and makes the liver and kidneys work harder. Doctors restrict protein intake when they put patients on a renal diet. Yet there is not much public awareness of this. Even as a nurse I knew this, but still, I did not question the hidden message of "more protein" that is in our culture. Most Americans eat *more* protein than their body needs because of messaging from the meat industry that pushes the importance of protein. The World Health Organization recommends about 5% of daily calories be eaten as protein. That comes out to be about thirty-eight grams for an active man and 29 grams for a woman. Much less than I had been consuming. Often, I would eat half my daily needs in a processed protein bar just as a snack between meals!

Animal protein has been shown to contribute to kidney disease and calcium loss. Research has also shown that several different foods can trigger inflammation, most notably dairy proteins. Eliminating these dairy products like milk, cheese, yogurt, and sour cream has been shown to help improve inflammation. Without fiber, animal protein stalls in our gut. Evidence links animal protein to chronic disease.

It is true that our bodies need protein, but not without other macronutrients like fat and carbohydrates. We need those to form the lipoproteins and glycoproteins created and used in our body. You can get all the protein you need to form these compounds with a plant-based diet. Not only that, - you will not suffer from excess protein on a whole food pant-based diet because whole plant foods naturally contain the amount of protein our bodies need. Plant-based protein does not stimulate acid production in our bodies in the same way animal protein does.

Spinach is 51% protein, beans 26% protein, oatmeal 16% protein, corn 12% protein, oatmeal 16% protein, corn 12% protein, potatoes 11% protein. Those are just a few plant protein sources. Complex carbohydrates in vegetables, fruits, oats, whole grains, brown rice, beans, & sweet potatoes, give a slow release of sugar and are also loaded with fiber which keeps our bowels moving.

The earlier you start good plant-based nutrition the bigger the impact it will have. The more meat children eat, the higher their cancer risk. Children as young as 8 years old are developing Type 2 diabetes. Nutrition also plays a role in asthma, allergies, acne, migraines, and ear infections. Protein needs peak in toddler years and then again in puberty - especially athletes. Kids need sufficient calorie intake. Serve them nutrient dense foods, including carbohydrates, in every meal to meet their needs.

I wish I knew when I was raising my children what I know now. I got some things right just by luck and circumstance. My kids ate vegetables well, but the milk and meat! For a long time, I thought we needed them for protein. Little did I know we were overeating protein. I also spent a lot of time wrongly believing fish and poultry were healthy meats as compared to red meat. Turns out the cholesterol content of muscle meat, red or white, is basically the same. Beef, pork, poultry, or seafood all have cholesterol. Even if fish and white meat were more healthy than red meat it does not mean they are healthy compared to plant-based proteins.

Now, just as with oil, I remember to ask, *"Compared to what?"*

Myth #8 "A vegan or vegetarian lacks many of the nutrients needed for good health."

Wrong. B12 is the only nutrient missing in eating plant-based foods. Vegans and vegetarians can get the B12 they need with fortified cereal or plant milk, fortified nutritional yeast, or a daily or weekly supplements or multivitamin containing B12. For an adult with normal absorption, a B12 dose of fifty microgram daily supplement OR 2000 microgram weekly supplement will prevent any deficiencies.

What is more, about one in three typical Americans, eating standard American fare are often short on B12 and other nutrients due to a lack of fruits and vegetables in their diet paired with an excess of alcohol consumption which impairs nutrient absorption. Therefore, many of us would benefit from supplements or regularly adding B12 fortified cereals, plant-based milks, or nutritional yeast to our meals. I have heard the old saying, "You are what you eat" more accurately stated, "You aren't just what you eat, you are what you absorb."

PART 2

Practice
Trust

**"You must always do the things
you think you cannot do."**

-Eleanor Roosevelt

CHAPTER SIX

Square One

Working with yourself
Makes life beautiful by Not
Making it ugly

Enough talk of wishes and goals. Here is where the plan gets put into action. One of the main barriers stopping people from taking control of their health is know-how. Part of the reason for this is because our culture has put such emphasis on experts. When we elevate others to expert status, we downgrade our abilities. Most lifestyle changes do not require and expert. Just come back to basic knowledge starting at square one:

You are responsible for activities you choose to participate in every day.
You are responsible for what you drink.
You are responsible for what goes into your mouth.
You are responsible for creating a space where you can relax and thrive.

You are responsible for getting enough rest.
You are responsible for keeping your space clean.

Trust yourself to take care of yourself. These are the life-style choices you use to impact health positively or negatively every day. Take care of your health and energy with good food, exercise, stress relief, family time, and sleep. Work with yourself to create an environment that supports your goals.

Making decisions ahead of time takes some stress off our brain. We are making decisions all the time throughout our day which leads to decision fatigue and bad decisions. For me, packing lunch is a good example of this. If I already have something nutritious along with me, when coworkers are ordering out for pizza as a group, it is easy to opt out. Or if I am on the road and have nutritious food packed for the ride, I am not as tempted to stop and eat less healthy options at a restaurant or fast-food place.

This chapter is going to sound repetitive. That is because there are not unique lifestyle changes for cancer and a different, special set for heart disease. It all overlaps as much of the disease we encounter in America, is lifestyle related. To treat or prevent it can be hard because changing habits takes time. On top of that, disease progression takes time. We have been taught to expect a pill to fix our ills. You may not want to be bothered by making lifestyle changes because in the beginning, symptoms may not seem so bad to put up with, but as these diseases progress, they can lead to more serious problems.

For instance,

- polycystic ovary syndrome can lead to infertility, menstrual dysfunction, and excess facial & body hair.
- Non-alcoholic fatty liver disease can lead to non-alcoholic steatohepatitis (NASH) which then leads

to liver fibrosis & cirrhosis, liver cancer, liver failure, and/or death.

- Diabetes can lead to nerve damage, amputations, eye damage, kidney failure, and/or death
- High blood pressure is known as the silent killer because often people with high blood pressure feel fine, yet we know over time it leads to poor health and risk of stroke and/or death
- Insulin resistance should also be addressed because it can lead to high blood pressure, heart disease, fatty liver disease, increased body fat, weight gain, and other chronic conditions.

I could go on about diseases that become worse. The point is, addressing health issues early is crucial to preventing future illness and disability. Yet in our current system we wait until disease is active to begin treatment. Furthermore, I cannot stress enough that many chronic diseases are interrelated. That is why they are called comorbidities.

The good news is lifestyle changes we make for one condition affect the other conditions that may also be present. Change in lifestyle habits can be scary, but change is happening one way or the other whether we like it or not. We might as well put a positive spin on it and take charge of what we are able to. There is a lot we can do to make a positive impact. Consider a brief overview of a few common debilitating diseases and you will see you already understand on a basic level how lifestyle choices can affect them.

Bowel Disease

A long, long time ago Hippocrates had the idea that, "All disease begins in the gut." He famously came up with the advice, "Let food be thy medicine."

It makes sense. When we eat, we are putting the outside world into our body. Except for oxygen, everything our body needs is absorbed from our digestive system. When we eat foods that supports our digestion, our digestion system supports us. Sleep, exercise, and stress also affect our bowels. Serotonin is made in our gut which affects our mood. You can naturally boost serotonin and reduce stress using the gut-brain connection and what you eat. When we exercise it increases the movement of food through our digestive system instead of having food sit for days in our bowels.

Overall, Americans repeatedly insult digestion with a diet high in sugary, high fat foods, excessive alcohol, multiple medicines (aspirin, ibuprofen, prescriptions medications including antibiotics), and a sedentary life. Caffeine also affects our digestion. Additionally, animal products change the bacteria in our gut and can cause constipation. We can improve the stomach pain, bloating, and nausea commonly caused by constipation by changing what we eat and moving more.

Fiber is magical. It can both soften stool, and it can bulk stool. More fiber in our diet leads to more diverse bacteria in our gut, which is a good thing. In absence of fiber in our diet bacteria in our gut start digesting the mucous layer of our intestine which leads to inflammation. Besides more regular bowel movements, fiber also helps fill us up leaving us satisfied for longer after a meal. Fiber can help regulate our blood sugar and lower cholesterol levels.

We support our digestion when we:

- Drink adequate water, - stay hydrated.
- Slowly introduce more fiber (most Americans don't eat enough) and decrease animal products
- Increase activity
- Decrease and eliminate alcohol and sugary foods
- Get adequate sleep and decrease stress

Fatigue

Fatigue can be the result of a combination of lifestyle choices: over-busy lives, not enough sleep, poor nutrition, and less exercise. Increased movement and better nutrition can both help with fatigue. Choosing to eat nutritious foods provides fuel our body needs to function. Exercise triggers endorphins that stimulate our minds.

Obviously, getting adequate sleep can help. When we sleep our brain is not sleeping. It is taking the time to reorganize information and memories. Sleep is essential to being awake. We spend about a third of our life asleep for that reason. Instead of feeling guilty about 8 hours of sleep, rejoice in the rejuvenation it provides for your body.

Going back to the gut. So often we eat more hours of the day than we sleep. There is growing evidence pointing to the importance of fasting to aid in cell repair while we sleep. I find when I cut off food for 12 hours at night, (7pm – 7am, 8 pm to 8am, or 9pm – 9am) I sleep more soundly and my internal alarm to wake up works better.

Choosing to do less busywork and add rest/down time to our day reduces fatigue, giving us more energy to enjoy our work and relationships.

Cancer

We are exposed to cancer causing carcinogens daily which trigger free radical release in our body. We need the antioxidants found only in plant-based foods to help fight them. On the other hand, animal products increase inflammation in our body. The clearer we can be about what food is healthy and what is not, the better off our health will be.

Studies have shown that animal proteins can promote cancer cell growth. Meat products change the bacteria in our gut which can lead to cancer. Insulin-like growth factor (which is found in dairy) has been shown to stimulate cancer cell growth. Eating plants provides our body with fiber and antioxidants which help protect against, neutralize, and fight cancer growth. Soy has been shown to have cancer preventing effects. Exercise has also been shown to reduce our risk for cancer.

When it comes to cancer the focus should be on nutrition education. Nutrition is a risk factor that we all can control. Colon cancer is the second biggest cancer killer in both men and women. We know it is associated with alcohol consumption, low fiber diets, sedentary lifestyle, and meat consumption. Those are things in our lifestyle which we can change ourselves. Headaches, upset stomach, and racing heart are thought to be caused by acetaldehyde produced by the liver when breaking down alcohol. Keep in mind acetaldehyde is known to cause cancer and is used in the production of plastic, glue, perfume, and more. So less alcohol seems logical for our livers' sake.

It has also been documented that breast cancer risk can also be reduced with lifestyle changes including increased exercise, decreased alcohol consumption, decreasing stress, eliminating smoking, decreased consumption of animal products, and eating more of the antioxidants only found in plants. Prostate cancer risk can also be reduced with lifestyle changes. Kidney cancer too has also been associated with lifestyle habits such as diet and smoking. Nitrosamines associated with kidney cancer are in cigarettes which are the same nitrosamines that are found in hot dogs, beef, chicken, and pork.

Changing what we eat and drink, avoiding toxins, and getting exercise are all things we are free to do daily to help reduce our cancer risks. Also, there are many herbal remedies and foods that you may have already heard have anti-cancer effects. Ginger, pepper, turmeric, blueberry, mushrooms, ginseng, noni, coconut, mistletoe, apricot kernel. Can there be side effects of herbal remedies? Yes, but think about the side effects of medications – especially chemotherapy!

Herbs can do what medications cannot. They can support the immune system while destroying cancer. Medications, on the other hand, destroy both the cancer AND the immune system. At the very least, it makes sense to use herbal remedies alongside chemotherapy to give the body support.

Alzheimer's/ Brain Health

Studies have shown decreased saturated and trans fatty acids in our diet can decrease risk for Alzheimer's. Eating plants with vitamin E and antioxidants found in nuts, seeds, grapes, strawberries, blueberries, and dark-skinned fruit (plums, cherries, apples) can improve mild memory dysfunction. Adequate hydration also promotes brain function. Other foods that may help prevent/treat impaired cognitive function are kimchi, vitamin C, vitamin E, peppers, celery, parsley, broccoli, spinach, cabbage, apple skin, pumpkin, and cantaloupe. Most of these foods are not weird or hard to find. They are readily available in fresh, canned, or frozen section of grocery stores waiting for you to buy them and take them home to eat.

Not only can you support your brain by eating nutrient dense plants, but you can also improve brain health with regular exercise. Cardiovascular exercise has been shown to improve brain function and mood, improve memory, and reverse brain shrinkage. Heat therapy such as a sauna or hot bath has been shown to have similar effects as exercise. Both have a positive impact on depression as well as cognition.

Other lifestyle choices also affect brain health. Managing stress and experiencing loving relationships have an impact on our mental and physical health. Avoiding alcohol can lead to overall improved cognitive function.

Liver Disease/Non-alcoholic Fatty Liver Disease (NAFLD)

It may seem like an oversimplification, but most liver disease is related to what we eat and drink, as was the case in the documentary "Super Size Me". Research inspired by the documentary went on to show that two fast-food meals a day for just one week led to decreased liver functions. NAFLD is now the most common chronic liver disease affecting 1 in 3 adults in the United States. It is well associated with the consumption of soft drinks and meat. Remember even one soda a day can substantially raise the odds of liver disease.

It is more well known that alcohol can injure the liver and lead to cirrhosis. Cirrhosis can lead to liver failure or liver cancer. Yet, as a society, we are just as careless in our consumption of alcohol as we are in our consumption of fast-food. Hepatitis, autoimmune disease, and toxins can also damage our liver. Like heart failure, you can live a long time with liver failure, but as it progresses it can be debilitating with bleeding disorders, fluid buildup, and fatigue.

When we eat meat, we get cholesterol overload which can lead to increased fat in the liver. The liver then tries to get rid of the excess cholesterol by dumping it back into the bloodstream. Also, when we eat fat, we increase the growth of bad bacteria in our gut which increases inflammation and causes loss of bacteria diversity in the gut. Our body needs cholesterol to function, HOWEVER, our body can make all the cholesterol it needs. When we eat eggs, meat, and dairy in our diet it increases fat in the liver, causes liver cell death & spilling contents into our blood which is indicated by increased liver enzyme blood tests. When our liver is unable to remove the extra cholesterol we eat in animal products, it builds up. The blood flows less easily and the body becomes fatter.

We can improve and prevent NAFLD and other disease by avoiding sugary and high cholesterol foods such as soda, eggs, meat, and dairy. On the bright side, like heart disease and other chronic diseases, early stages of fatty liver disease, can be improved with lifestyle changes.

Kidney Disease

Kidneys filter our blood. Similar to the liver, toxic overload from what we eat and drink can lead to kidney failure.

Overeating protein can hurt our kidneys. Most Americans eat more protein than their body needs because we are continually urged to remember the importance of protein. There is a lack of awareness of what kidney failure treatment looks like. Let me be clear that dialysis is not a walk in the park. A person does not just have dialysis and go on with their merry life. It is time consuming and often comes with complications, debilitation, and fatigue. Often these patients are so exhausted between treatments that they have little energy to do anything except rest between treatments.

Organ transplants are not an easy answer either. For starters, transplant is not a given. There has to be an organ available that is compatible. Beyond that, transplants surgeries are invasive with risks and recovery time. I have taken care of patients in both scenarios. Either scenario makes not over-eating protein seem like a worthwhile exchange to decrease our risk of kidney disease. In addition, we can lessen our risk for kidney disease with other lifestyle habits: drink plenty of fluids, avoiding excessive caffeine or sugary drinks, avoid added salt, and eat a variety of fruits and vegetables.

The same recommendations hold true for decreasing our risk for kidney stones. Kidney stones are becoming more common and for years have been linked to increased animal protein consumption while those with higher intake of fruits and vegetables have been shown to have a reduced risk of kidney stones. It is thought to have to do with the acid producing effect of animal protein consumption causing acid build up that was previously discussed in the myth busting section versus the alkalizing effect of some fruits and vegetables.

Polycystic Ovary Syndrome (PCOS)

PCOS is associated with dietary intake of Advanced Glycation End Products (AGEs). It is thought that because AGEs receptors are concentrated in the ovaries, they contribute to PCOS.

Ways to improve/prevent PCOS:

1. Avoid smoking
2. Decrease high AGEs foods (meat, cheese, and eggs cooked at high temps i.e. broiled, grilled, fried, & roasted)
3. Increase foods that help pull AGEs out of system like brown rice & mushrooms

4. Increase foods with antioxidants like berries, herbs, and spices
5. Change method of cooking from high dry heat (broiling, searing, frying) to low heat with high humidity (stewing, steaming, boiling)

Studies have shown making these kinds of changes can show improvement of PCOS in as little as 2 months.

Diabetes or Borderline Diabetes

About 1 in 3 Medicare dollars is spent on diabetes in the US. Diabetes is the seventh leading cause of death, and it begins with insulin resistance. Fat in our diet causes insulin resistance which can lead to type two diabetes. Studies dating back almost one hundred years ago observed elevated glucose intolerance in those eating a high fat diet versus those eating a high carbohydrate diet. Fat we eat can build up in cells making it hard for sugar to move from our blood stream into our cells. People think high sugar is the problem, but the problem is the fat buildup that is preventing the sugar from entering cells by blocking insulin. The fat is gumming up the lock that insulin uses to allow sugar in. No matter how much insulin is in the blood, glucose cannot get into our muscle. Then fatty muscle leads to fatty liver which leads to a fatty pancreas which eventually gives out from the overwork of producing insulin that the body cannot use because of the fat in our bloodstream.

The fat in our bloodstream comes from the saturated fat we eat and the fat in our bodies. When fat cells in our body become too full, they spill over into the bloodstream. They also activate an inflammatory response and create a vicious cycle. Diets high in processed foods and animal products contribute to increased fat in the body. (Also, animal protein has been shown to contribute to kidney disease and calcium loss.) As I mentioned before, the popular treatment of a high-fat, low-carbohydrate diet can cause *more* insulin resistance which could be why we are seeing our incidence of diabetes going up, not down. It is not publicized well, but research instead points to a low-fat, plant-based, whole-food diet which includes natural carbohydrates such as those in sweet potatoes, carrots, corn, and whole grains.

Most of us understand processed sugars are not a friend to our health. Refined sugars can negatively affect our teeth, our gum, and inflammation in our body. Swap out added sugars for fruit. The human body treats sugar in fruit different than refined sugars. Apples, bananas, berries, peaches, grapefruit, and oranges come not just with sugar, but with fiber so you do not get the sugar crash. People living in Blue Zones eat whole foods containing carbohydrates and they do not have the incidence of diabetes America has. Our avoidance of healthy carbohydrates found in fruits and vegetables does nothing to address the fat that is blocking the ability of sugar to be used. What our avoidance does is cause us to miss out on healing antioxidants found in these foods.

We can address that fat by adjusting what we eat. A diagnosis of type 2 diabetes does not have to mean a lifetime of medicine and shots. People can make choices in their lifestyle to get in a little activity, take care of their relationships, and make the following nutrition choices.

Ways to improve/prevent DM with nutrition:

1. Fill your plate with whole grains, legumes, fruits, and vegetables.
2. Cut back on processed carbohydrates such as refined sugar and white flour products.
3. Cut animal products such as meat, cheese, and dairy from your plate.

4. Avoid added oils and other high fat plant foods (vegetable oil, olive oil, corn oil, coconut oil, etcetera… and *excess* nuts, seeds, & avocados)
5. For a sweet treat slice up a piece of fruit like an apple, a pear or a peach. Try frozen berries or other frozen fruit.

Insulin resistance is not just impacted by the food we eat. Genetic history, lack of exercise, or excessive alcohol intake also play a role. Combining regular exercise with good nutrition helps to burn excess fat stores and reverse insulin resistance. With consistent exercise your body will begin burning fat stores even faster with the afterburn effect. We cannot change our genetic history, but we can change the habits that affect the way our genes are expressed.

Chronic Inflammation/ Autoimmune Disease/ Pain

Inflammation is at the root of chronic disease. Research has shown that several different foods can trigger inflammation, most notably dairy proteins. Eliminating dairy products like milk, cheese, yogurt, and sour cream has been shown to help improve inflammation. Foods high in refined sugar, for example, those in baked goods, snack foods, and sugary beverages, are also known to be inflammatory. Red meats have also been shown to trigger inflammation and cause autoimmune disease flare up.

It is logical to avoid those foods known to cause inflammation and consume those known to decrease inflammation (think antioxidants) such as (but not limited to) cruciferous vegetables, berries, and turmeric/curcumin.

Increased movement can help support surrounding muscles and bones for better mobility and decreased pain.

Overweight and Obesity

We have unprecedented levels of people with weight control issues in America right now.

As previously addressed, one of greatest myths of modern day is that if we just move more, we will lose weight. Eating a low-fat diet is a better place to start. Fat has five more calories per gram than either carbohydrates or protein. Oil provides 4,000 calories per pound which is forty times more calories than a pound of fruits or vegetables. Decreasing the fat we eat can help decrease our weight.

Cutting animal meat and dairy will reduce the amount of fat on your plate. White meat, like chicken, is promoted as being healthy, but about a quarter of the calories of a skinless piece comes from fat. Our intensive agriculture practices have purposely increased the amount of fat in poultry. Avoid adding oil to food and avoid processed foods with oil of any type in the ingredient list. Watch labels carefully as oil is added unnecessarily into plant milks and other manufactured vegan foods or "health" foods.

Eating fat in our foods simultaneously with carbohydrates allows our body to burn the carbohydrate and store the fat. For instance, a baked potato with butter or a baked potato with a steak is a carb/fat combo that leads to weight gain. Baked goods with sugar and added oil are another example of carbohydrate/fat combo that should be avoided.

Increased fiber from plant foods helps fill us up while displacing other unhealthy foods. Fiber also helps carry fat out of our body during digestion. It also binds with other toxins to carry them out of our body. Beans, broccoli, rice, oatmeal, orange, banana, and whole grains are all fiber rich foods that help prevent weight gain.

Another myth around being overweight is if we eat less, we will lose weight. We often put a lot of focus on managing portion sizes. It is possible to eat large portions if we pay closer attention to what we are eating. We can fill our plate with beans, vegetables, & whole grains without animal products and added oils to increase our fiber intake and decrease our calorie intake while still eating large, satisfying quantities that fill us up.

A benefit of good nutrition is more energy to exercise. Exercise *with* good nutrition is a much more effective recipe for weight loss than exercise alone to make up for bad nutrition. Also, cardiovascular exercise is known to affect energy levels and even sexual performance. Eat for better performance and movement. This change in mindset goes a long way in maintaining a healthy body weight.

High Blood Pressure/Heart Disease

I am sure you know your heart circulates blood through your body, but do you ever think why that is important? Our blood is transporting oxygen, nutrients, and hormones that our cells need. Each heartbeat requires the compounds and chemicals our heart is circulating. Besides carrying oxygen and nutrients to the cells that line our blood vessels, these nutrients also help keep neighboring cells healthy. As blood pressure goes up, so does our risk for heart attack or stroke. So, we want to maintain a pressure that is supportive of the needs of the body.

Amino acids found in plants increase our body's ability to regulate nitric oxide and keep blood vessels healthy. Saturated fat in animal meat and dairy products makes the blood move more slowly. We know oil moves slower than water. It is the same with fatty blood versus low-fat blood. Fat in our blood also affects the lining of our blood vessels making it harder for blood to flow through.

Animal products provide cholesterol in our diets that leads to heart disease. Eggs are the food highest in cholesterol. Saturated fat in animal meats prompts our body to produce extra cholesterol. Fat to avoid includes foods with plant oils: olive oil, grapeseed oil, palm oil, coconut oil. All oils can harm our cardiovascular system.

Cholesterol is a fat-like waxy substance found in your blood and body's cells. Cholesterol is only found in animals. Our bodies create cholesterol as they need it. When we eat cholesterol, our body makes more cholesterol. In this way, when you eat animal-based foods you are taking on excess amounts of cholesterol. There are two types of cholesterol. Low-density lipoprotein (LDL - the "bad" cholesterol) and high-density lipoprotein (HDL - the "good" cholesterol). LDL is commonly referred to as "the bad" cholesterol and HDL as "the good" cholesterol.

LDL can build up in the inner walls of arteries and form plaques which narrow the vessels. The lower the number your LDL, the better. Elevated levels can cause high blood pressure and put you at increased risk for stroke and/or heart attack.

Anxiety can increase blood pressure.

Caffeine and alcohol are stimulants that can contribute to high blood pressure.

Fiber in plants can help carry unwanted cholesterol out of our body through digestion. Oatmeal, soy, and nuts can help lower cholesterol too. We can also eat for nitric oxide. Nitric oxide is important for heart function because it helps keep our blood vessels relaxed. Eating greens helps promote nitric oxide in our body to protect blood vessel lining and prevent it from becoming sticky. Preventing stickiness prevents buildup of cholesterol in our blood vessels.

Sodium content in processed foods like cheese, lunch-meat, and canned soups can also contribute to high blood pressure. Choosing plant foods that are naturally lower in sodium and higher in potassium helps to lower blood pressure. Maintaining a healthy weight can improve our blood pressure. Lack of sleep and stress can also affect our blood pressure. Exercise can help decrease our blood pressure, improve sleep, and reduce stress. Cardiovascular disease is related to inflammation as much as elevated cholesterol and blood pressure. So, we should not underestimate how these lifestyle changes also help to decrease inflammation in our body which can be seen with improving inflammatory marker lab tests.

Blood pressure can be impacted or prevented with these long-accepted lifestyle interventions:

- Eat Healthy: Low salt, low sugar, low fat
- Maintain a healthy weight
- Do not smoke or chew tobacco products
- Get adequate exercise
- Limit alcohol
- Manage stress levels
- Effectively manage chronic conditions (if you have them) such as diabetes or elevated cholesterol

While measuring blood pressure can be helpful in tracking your health, getting too focused on numbers is sometimes counterproductive. Your blood pressure can change from minute to minute. Focus on looking for *trends* in your pressure.

CHAPTER SEVEN

Whole, Big, Delicious Life

Come as you are friend
Now the choice is yours to make
Hurry - don't be late!

Now that we have looked closer at some common preventable diseases, we can see the common underlying lifestyle choices that impact them. Gather what you need for the recipe. Then make the decision to start following the recipe for a big, delicious life. Being more mindful about the choices we make regarding food, activity, and stress can have a huge impact on many areas of our physical and mental health.

These are the measures we are implementing into our lifestyle to create health. This is the recipe for a big, delicious life:

1. Get proper rest
2. Nurture our mind & relationships

3. Eat a whole food plant-based diet, - low in sugar, salt, and fat - stay hydrated
4. No smoking & limit alcohol
5. Be Active

On a basic level we know that each of these measures are good for our health. Eating fruits and vegetables is good for us. What we might not realize is that we can get all the nutrients we need from eating just sweet potatoes alone. It does not have to be complicated. If we are eating a variety of good nutritious vegetables, we can rest assured that we will be meeting our nutritional requirements for fat, carbohydrates, and protein. We know that increased activity helps build strength and balance in our movement. We know connecting with others helps our emotional well-being. We know we function better after a nap or good night's rest. We can tell that smoking and alcohol affects our mood, judgement, and physical abilities.

Focus on the *actions you are taking* to keep your body healthy and strong. Focus on the new skills you are gaining. No experts needed. We got this!

To keep yourself accountable, track your progress. One of the ways I started was with a simple activity tracker with my most important things on it. From your chapter four goals, take the one that you feel is the most important and focus on it. Start a habit around it so that you can be true to yourself and know you are doing what you can for your health. Consider using an app. If you are using a digital activity tracker, they often give information on heartrate and sleep too. If expense, privacy, or learning tech is a concern, tracking your habits can be as simple as using a piece of paper or marking it on a calendar. Nowadays, I keep track right on my weekly panner, so everything is in one place.

A journal also helped me to lead with my values. Putting pen to paper helps me to recognize projects (or work) that are exhilarating but create stress by conflicting with my values. A journal can help to focus on being resilient and learning to align values with your work and life. Many activity trackers allow for journaling about mood and food intake all in the same app.

Personally, I prefer a planner that allows room for notes & journaling for each week, so everything is in the same place, and I do not have to worry about internet connections or syncing. I do use apps and devices, but most of my tracking is on paper.

Obviously, we will still want to learn the main skills and subskills for each area. While we are learning it is important to recognize when we encounter "disinformation/misinformation" that creates confusion. This is different than the fish out of water confusion that is normal with learning new skills. We can learn the lifestyle skills on our own by just jumping in and self-correcting as needed. We cannot always turn to government, business, or other individual gurus to help us. Often, they have a financial conflict of interest which prevents them from having our health as their primary concern.

We must start with looking to ourselves for the answers to our health. Nobody knows our body better than we know it. Continually seeking information from proclaimed gurus and experts leads to more confusion. Once we take it upon ourselves to get start with a tracker or journal, we gain momentum to build on.

Get proper rest

Eight hours of sleep per night for an adult seems to be an accepted standard. Creating a bedtime routine and creating boundaries around our sleep can go a long way in helping us get those eight hours. Everyone is different. Pay attention to how many hours seems to feel best for you. You may do better on seven or nine.

Our body follows a cycle: sleep helps support our activity through the day then our movement through the day helps support our sleep. Sleep is a key ingredient for cellular repair. It helps our body organize our mind to tackle the next day.

One of the first things I began supporting was my sleep. I had spent years working night shifts and my on/off cycles were wrecked. I knew sleep was a base for energy, but I had long since removed rituals and boundaries around it. There were many mornings I would be too tired to drive home and would have to pull over to sleep an hour or two. Then I would wake up, get home, and sleep another couple of hours. It was not a great way to get up feeling rested.

On nights when I did not work, I still did not allow myself an "off" button. If there was work around the house to be done, I kept going: sweep floors, clean bathrooms, fold laundry. Or I would watch television with the kids taking in all the built-in advertising that goes along with it: beer commercials, food ads, commercials selling the latest gizmo, etc. Not exactly good quality time for any of us. It was not until much later that I discovered the idea that at the end of the day I can allow myself to stop being productive and just enjoy time alone or with my family. It is okay if I start to feel tired in the evening. That means I have been up all day and my body is telling me it is time to think about winding down for sleep.

It is good to learn to recognize when we are feeling tired. Taking time during the day for a rest period can be as simple as listening to soft music. Sit down and phone a friend for a chat. Read an article or chapter in a book. Take a catnap. Sometimes a slow stroll outside in fresh air for five or ten minutes can help us feel more energized. Breathe in the fresh air and relax. Just because we are tired does not mean we cannot take a brief walk. I have found when I focus too much on productivity, I end up sleep deprived. It has taken some doing, but I am better at gauging my energy levels and taking time out to "smell the roses," rest, and enjoy what it is I am being productive for in the first place.

In the beginning my basic goal was to get six to seven hours of continuous sleep at night. I started to set my sleep and wake times. I was in bed by midnight and up at six or in bed by eleven and up at five. I began to feel better and now I aim for 7 to 8 hours of sleep at night. If my work schedule changes, I adjust my bedtime accordingly.

If you are not getting enough sleep start by watching your weekday bedtimes. Then when weekends come - watch out! Lack of sleep on weekends can throw off your rhythm for the rest of the week. Try to keep your sleep and wake times consistent even on weekends. If you are way off your current goal, try just adding one more hour at a time until gradually you get where you feel rested. Remember this is not about being rigid. We simply want *most* nights to provide adequate rest.

Caffeine does not seem to affect my sleep as much, but I notice alcohol does. In the past, when I had a beer or glass of wine close to bedtime, I was restless waking up a few times through the night. I still occasionally have coffee in the afternoon or at dinner, but most days I try to limit any caffeine to morning hours. I used to drink about three pots of coffee in a 24-hour period. Now some days I do not have any. Now that I am sleeping properly, I am not relying on caffeine to keep me going. Alcohol was harder because if I had a drink, it was usually in the evening. Spacing it at least two hours before bedtime seemed to help keep it from disrupting my sleep. Overall, I do better if I avoid it completely. I wake up in a better mood and without any heaviness when I do not drink alcohol.

Last year, I gave up alcohol for a year as a New Year's Resolution. This year instead of going back to alcohol I have tried a few non-alcohol beers and wine which have had good flavor and work if I feel incline to have a beer. The replacements I found throughout last year for a glass of wine or a cold beer suit me fine. Instead of caffeine or alcohol in the evening, I find herbal tea like chamomile relaxing. Giving up alcohol for a year also gave me the knowledge that I can live just fine without alcohol.

What is not relaxing for me is clutter. This is a problem because I have always been a bit of a pack rat. My bedroom often turns into a "catch all" of items that accumulate throughout the week. Taking time to try to keep my bedroom orderly makes it a more relaxing space to rest. A cool room with clean sheets and no clutter helps set the stage for a good night's sleep.

Another strategy I used to get more sleep was to establish a wind down routine. Once the kitchen is cleaned up after dinner, I turn off the overhead lights and turn on softer lamps. I may watch some of the evening news or a television show, but then I try to stop any device screen time too close to bed. Taking time for changing into pajamas, washing face, and brushing teeth helps fill that time before bed and cue my body that it is time for sleep. Sometimes I listen to music or diffuse essential oils to create a calming mood. Often I read.

As far as my phone is concerned, I do best when I have it set to go into sleep mode an hour before bed. Studies have shown phones are less addicting when in greyscale. When the screen goes to black and white, I am less likely to fiddle with it. I have made it a habit to be low-tech from 10pm to 7am. On good nights I place my phone out of reach so that if I do wake up in the middle of the night, I do not check it.

I like to have a pen and paper at my bedside in case I cannot sleep. I write down what is on my mind so that I can let it go. Another way to wind down for bed is to celebrate the day. Some researchers claim what you think about the final 30 minutes before sleep replays in your head 15-17 times while you sleep. So, if before you turn out the light, you make a special effort to think of the positive moments of the day that will be played over and over and dominate your sleep rather than any anxieties or worries you may have.

Taking time for deep breathing can also help your body relax before sleep. A simple technique is taking an inhalation for 4 seconds, hold it for 2 seconds, and then exhale for 7 seconds. This 4-2-7 deep breathing technique can be used any time of day but repeating it a few times before bed can be a calming part of winding down. Guided imagery can also be helpful. I prefer to simply review a relaxing part of my day or imagine a relaxing past vacation day or moment as I breathe deeply to reset my mind before sleep. It also helps reset my body as deep breathing is known to decrease blood pressure and heart rate.

The rituals we create around sleep help us to get the rest we need to restore our body physically. It also helps us mentally and emotionally. Bedtime rituals are also a good time to connect with those we live with. A good night's sleep helps us wake up to face the day with clarity, focus, and more energy. When you reach a point when you wake up refreshed before your alarm goes off, congratulations! That is a sign you had a good night's sleep.

Nurture our mind and relationships

Our relationships with others have been linked to adding years to our life, wellness, and disease prevention. When we connect and play with others, we understand each other better and reduce stress and inflammation. Not only that, but it is also fun! As you make changes to your lifestyle avoid fighting with others about it. These types of arguments are a pitfall.

Instead connect with others by taking time to listen to them and what they are concerned about in their life.

Forgiveness can be a key component that has a positive impact on our mind and relationships.

There are different situations in our life that call for us to open our hearts to someone we value who has hurt us, realizes it, apologizes, and is sorry. Then there are other situations where we have been violated and the person or people are not sorry. If needed, you can even forgive yourself for mistakes you may have made it the past. Resentment festers in our hearts and minds, drains our energy, and keeps us from carrying on with our life. Some wrongs can never be righted. What happens in the past happened in the past. Let it go with forgiveness to heal yourself and allow yourself to move forward and flourish. Studies have shown forgiveness can improve our physical health decreasing risk for heart attack, reducing pain and blood pressure, and decreasing depression, anxiety, and stress.

Supportive relationships with those we love and trust, reduce our stress and improve our coping skills during times of struggle. Other people matter in our lives as they give us an opportunity to tell our story and reminisce on shared moments. They also help us make changes if needed and move forward in new directions. Our success in health and in life is dependent on how well we get along with the people around us. Learning to accept that we can control only our own behavior goes a long way in freeing us from unhealthy relationships. At the same time, we know our behaviors affect the lives of those around us. Just as we determine what freedoms we are willing to give up for the sake of the relationship, we determine what we are willing to contribute to a relationship. Other people can be a source of positive feedback loops for us, just as we can be a source of positive feedback for them.

We talked about deep breathing to relax before sleep. Deep breathing can also be helpful whenever you start to feel anxious or mad in a relationship. I try to keep my head, so I am putting my best foot forward and setting up the relationship for others to do the same.

Eat a whole food plant-based diet, - low in sugar, salt, and fat.

Getting good nutrition for your body to be healthy means avoiding mindless intake of too many calories. Be aware of added oil. It bears repeating. In calories per pound of food, fruits and vegetables are 60 to 420 calories per pound while added oil is 4,000 calories per pound. That is a huge difference! You get *more food* with *less calories* when you eat plant-based options, and you feel more satisfied because your stomach is fuller.

If we pay attention, most of us can acknowledge that we are surrounded by unhealthy high calorie, fat, salt, and sugar filled food choices. In America there is a disconnect between our food supply and our medical care. *We are perfectly willing to believe medicine that we swallow will help heal us, yet we fight the idea that the food that we swallow is making us sick.* There are many diets out there that can be successful for weight loss, but weight loss does not necessarily equal health. You will find that simply saying you are vegan or going keto does not automatically do the trick to gain better health. There are plenty of junk food vegans who are not healthy. Eat more low-calorie vegetables, fruits, potatoes, beans, and whole grains than you do higher calorie breads, sugars, dry cereals, chips, crackers, nuts, seeds, and added oils. When we eat foods that have less calories per pound, we can eat big portions and still lose weight or maintain our weight, depending on our activity and goals.

When we are just starting out, we might have a goal to eat one or two real vegetables a day. Maybe you want to try two meatless dinners per week. When I began eating more fruits and vegetables, I started with breakfast. Then I moved on to lunch and dinner. Many times, my lunch is leftovers from dinner the previous day, so my progress moved along faster than I expected. Another goal when I began, was to eliminate all soda and sugary drinks which eventually included "health" smoothies with added sugar and protein powders. Now when I make a smoothie, I stick with whole food ingredients. The more we choose to pass up unhealthy options the more momentum we build and eventually the healthy choices begin to outweigh the junk and fast-food.

No smoking and limit alcohol

I almost did not include this on my list because I did not want anyone to disregard the rest simply because they got stuck here. For a long time, smoking was considered fashionable, and that is coming back among young people with vaping today. At the same time, there are obvious unpleasant side effects of smoking such as smokers cough and shortness of breath. Studies have shown smoking is not healthy for our lungs and blood vessels.

Alcohol, on the other hand, has remained fashionable despite being unhealthy. If you have ever seen someone who has had too much to drink, you may have noticed how alcohol impairs their speech and coordination. Sometimes they cannot even function with appropriate conversations. Their speech can be loud, slurred, and/or rambling. Their reaction time and coordination are decreased impairing activities or work that require it. Research has shown how alcohol negatively affects our liver, brain, and digestive system. Yet it continues to be part of the rite of passage in America of a child into adulthood.

What I dislike most about tobacco and alcohol is their addictive nature. I would rather not have a chemical influencing me to continually consume something harmful to my body and relationships. I do not like the idea of others profiting from my demise either. If you smoke or drink alcohol there are many cessation programs to choose from. This is an area where asking for help can be a benefit. I know people who have quit on their own too. Before anyone quits, they must want to do it for themselves. An A-team is important to lift us when we falter, but only we can make the choice for ourselves of what we put into our body.

Caffeine and alcohol drinks can dehydrate. Drinks are often a source of empty calories. Switching to water, infused with lemon or fruit for a hint of flavor, or caffeine free herbal tea will provide better hydration. Use a reusable bottle that you can easily track that you are drinking an adequate amount of liquid daily.

Be Active

Renewed energy is what helps us to work and play. Life is a mental game as much as anything. Sometimes we find ourselves in a slump. We do not know how we got there, and we do not know how to get out. Then just as suddenly something clicks, and we are back in the game. It seems to me the key is in moving forward. Just because there were dropped balls, strikeouts, and missed opportunities in the last inning, does not mean the team can't come back in the next inning, score five runs, and take the lead to win the game.

It is the days of consistency that help carry us through days that are not so good. We already know that we have the capability of having good days because we have had them in the past. The more days we have where we get rest, eat nutritious food, and exercise, the less days that do not go as planned set us back. Eating a piece of cake is not the end of the world. Just as skipping four days of walking does not mean we quit altogether. Just jump back in where you left off.

Focusing on the big picture and our purpose can empower us to deal better with bumps in the road. Not only does it make us more resilient it can improve the quality of our relationships and our overall satisfaction with life. We are wired for survival, and we do hard things on a regular basis. It is our purpose and the light at the end of the tunnel gets us through it.

If you think you can, you give yourself a chance. Now is a good time to start rituals that make fitness a priority in your lifestyle. Do not ruminate on what you have done in the past. Everyone can show a little grit and work with adding some activity into the day. Remember the activities you listed in chapter 3? Use those as you begin to take steps to add activities and adventure to your life. Some activities are simpler than others, but they all start with taking the first step. Think of what you can do at home or close to home with minimal equipment. What can you do that uses your natural abilities? That may be a walk, go to the park, go to a gym and workout, play basketball, or jump rope. The possibilities are endless. As we increase our physical activity, we will find our sleep improving. Laying out clothes, shoes, and a jacket to cue ourselves to take a morning walk can help us stick with an activity plan rather than giving in to our mood in the moment. The momentum of taking the first steps leads to more action.

We get more of what we nurture. We must show up for what we want even when we do not feel like it. I have been on 3-day kickstarts, 21-day challenges, 10-day jumpstarts and they all start out the same way. I am excited and enthusiastic, but if I do not plan to fit the new program or information into the day then they soon get lost in the shuffle. So before beginning, set yourself up for success by planning to give the activity the time it requires.

We were designed to be outside, be active, and be social. If you have become more sedentary or are stuck in a chair all day for work, a starter goal might be just to get outside and move for 10 minutes three times a day. If you are put off by the word exercise rephrase it in your mind into something more enjoyable. *I am going to go outside to look at the flowers in the park and see if there are any ducks on the pond after lunch.* The important thing is to decide when, where and with who you are going to move with and plan for it.

I am using "after lunch" as an example because when I first started adding movement to my day, I would meet a couple of friends after lunch and walk around our office building. This was time I would otherwise have worked through even though I still had time I was "allowed" to be away from my desk. The ideal time to plan more movement in your day is when you can trade time you might normally spend on distractions, unhelpful habits, or addictions. Think where in your day you can swap out an activity that is not supporting your health for movement that is. Also think about times of the day when you have the most energy and your intention will be strong.

If you have a dog (or a friend with a dog) sometimes taking the dog for a walk can be a good reason to be active. It is good for you and good for the dog. Depending on what your goals are, keeping it fun and playful inspires you to want to do it again. Make it easy and enjoyable. The easier you make it the more likely you are to stick with it. If you enjoy it, you will feel more satisfied.

Another way I stay motivated to move is signing up for an event like a charity walk or run. When we build friendships with others who are interested in the same things, we are creating a support system for each other. You could join or start a walking group.

Moving with friends also gives us that built-in feedback loop to evaluate our progress. We can use a pedometer or device activity tracker for feedback too. I often keep a simple chart on my calendar and place a star or check mark on days I get my exercise in. Some days I work harder than others and at times I am building progression with varying intensities to meet a bigger goal. It is important to listen to my body and not overdo it. While I move more another goal overall is to avoid injury. I do not always push as hard as I could, but to me it is more important to have fun and not hurt myself than to be competitive. I do not want to take myself out of the game with an injury that I could avoid by not overusing or overstressing my body.

If you are moving while doing something you are good at, you are exercising. That makes you an athlete. We do not have to be competitive to be good at physical exercise. If you want to take it to the next level, go for it! Compete in an event that requires more than what I am talking about here. For this book, I am simply promoting creating a lifestyle that allows for activity and movement to be a part of your daily routine. Either way, consistency with activity gets us the results we want.

Building relationships around exercise can help establish activity habits. If you have a friend to walk and talk with it helps you connect while at the same time, be active. Moving more is not just about how we look and having a toned-up body. Increased activity improves our mood and how our body functions.

Doing a variety of exercise supports our body in different ways. Cardiovascular exercise elevates your heart rate and breathing. It improves the performance of our heart and lungs which improves the flow of oxygen and nutrients through our body. Strength training benefits by increasing muscle strength and endurance. These exercises also help us with balance, increase bone density, and help prevent osteoporosis and joint injuries. Increasing our flexibility with exercise such as yoga, also helps prevent injury. Plus, stretching exercises improve our balance and posture, and increase our mobility and coordination. Yoga helps with mind body connection and our connection with the world and others.

Most of this is common knowledge. We have the knowledge but are not putting it to use. Other barriers we suppose are in our way are family, money, time, and availability. Money spent on hobbies can add up, but there are lots of activities that are free. Taking a walk in the morning, at lunch time or after dinner does not cost anything. Going for a run or jog is free. You do not need to join a gym. Basic calisthenics, body weight exercises, and yoga do not require any special equipment or a gym membership. Just because there are many options for us to spend money on exercise and activity – join a gym, hire a trainer, buy fancy clothes or gear – does not mean we have to.

When we say we do not have time, we don't have the money, or it is not available, what we are really saying is that it isn't important to us. It is not in our quality world. We choose what is important and what and who we spend time and money on.

It may surprise you to find that living a healthy lifestyle is quite affordable. I remember years ago taking care of a patient who was a three pack per day cigarette smoker. He was sick in the hospital for a couple of weeks. During that time, he began to calculate how much money he had been spending on cigarettes which added up to thousands of dollars a year. He began to realize he was wasting money on products that harmed his health. You may think that should have been obvious to him, but the same can be said for money spent on beer, wine, and potato chips. Millions of us are doing the same thing daily. We are spending money on products that are making us sick.

Eating healthy is *eating simple*. It is so simple that it is eluding us. Simple food is picked off a tree or grown out of the ground. Despite their simplicity, they are packed with nutrients. These simple foods are less expensive than processed products and less expensive than animal products. Frozen or fresh produce, beans, rice, potatoes, and whole grain or gluten free pasta are readily available and are some of the cheapest items in the grocery store. When eating out, often dishes without meat are less expensive than those that include it. Buying in bulk or by the case is another way to make simple foods affordable.

We take the time to sit in a fast-food line. We find the money to buy alcohol or cigarettes. We have the money to buy the latest technology. We take the time to shop for the new game or shoes we want. Yet we do not take time to find which restaurants serve whole healthy foods. We do not take time to go outside for a walk in the morning before work or on our break.

We know more than we give ourselves credit for about disease. Without others telling us, we understand how lifestyle impacts our health. America is a rich country. We have the money for, and the availability of, products at our fingertips twenty-four hours a day. Why is the overall health of our communities decreasing?

We can stop allowing others to make choices for us. We can stop allowing others to mislead us with confusing campaigns. We can choose to move more. We can choose to eat more nutritious foods. We can choose to nurture our minds and our relationships. We choose what we focus on, what we spend our money on, and what we spend our time doing.

We do not have to be experts to take the next step, evaluate our progress, and keep learning. Take a deep breath and keep moving. We have resources. We do not have to be certain of all the answers. We just need to be willing to do the work and have an open heart and mind to keep moving forward.

As we move forward another common constraint that may present itself as a stumbling block is family and friends. We cannot very well leave them out of the picture since they are on this journey with us. You may have noticed that relationships can be present in all the lifestyle areas. Our sleep, exercise, and food rituals can all involve friends, family, and community. When those around us notice us making changes in our lifestyle they may give some push back. They may not want to be left behind. They may be worried about how the changes will affect them. The best I have been able to do is to assure people I am not expecting them to make the same changes and I try to assure them and show them that I am "still me." I try to let them know I am just letting go of things that are not healthy for me. Some people get it. Some people do not.

While some people may not want to have anything to do with lifestyle changes that affect what they have been eating and doing for years, there are bound to be a few people in your life who "get it" and are supportive of your goals. It is important to make sure you have at least a few conversations a day where you feel heard and understood. That goes for life in general, not just regarding exercise, rest, and eating for health.

Our relationships are part of our health. If you feel you do not have people in your life where there is a good balance of give and take, now is the time to build some. Start looking for spaces in your community where you can be yourself and have good conversations. That does not mean you have to ditch your friends and family and normal hangouts. It just means you are adding other people and places to your life for support.

We can use that same mentality when thinking of food, exercise, and rest too. It is not that we cannot watch tv or play video games. We get to go outside for a walk. It is not that we cannot eat donuts and hamburgers. We *get to choose healthy* foods that help our body function at its best. We are *adding in* all good things to build an environment that helps us flourish.

CHAPTER EIGHT

Week One

The moment is now
That's enough preparation
Put it in practice

Water

General rule of thumb for staying hydrated is drink half your body weight in ounces of water daily.

General rule of thumb for staying hydrated is drink half your body weight in ounces of water daily.

For instance:

If you weigh 100 pounds drink 50 ounces of water daily
If you weigh 130 pounds drink 65 ounces of water daily
If you weigh 150 pounds drink 75 ounces of water daily
If you weigh 200 pounds drink 100 ounces of water daily

Add more for hot weather, increased physical activity, or strenuous exercise.

Try using a graduated water bottle to track your fluid intake.

Try to avoid even smoothies and juices at this point. Focus on chewing fruits and vegetables and turning to plain, old water for hydration.

Sleep

General sleep recommendations are 8 hours per night. Children and teens may require more. Sleep for adults varies. Find what works for your body to feel rested.

General sleep recommendations are 8 hours per night.

Is your sleep space clean, safe, and quiet? Do what you can to create a clean environment for sleep. Get rid of clutter and snuggle up in clean bed linens. Take any extra measures so that you feel safe when you are sleeping. I sometimes wear ear plugs or an eye mask if noise or lights from others are an issue.

If you have not already, consider what kind of a wind down routine could help to cue your body and mind that it is time to rest. Brushing our teeth, putting on pajamas, and washing our face can all be signals to our brain that we are getting ready to rest.

Activity

Walking and running are two activities that most humans can do without much thought. Just because they can be effortless does not mean they cannot be used to build function, strength, and endurance. Also, it is something you can do at home or close to home in your neighborhood. While we are adding activity remember that we want to displace previous habits or addictions we identified in Part One. Make it more difficult to spend time on these old activities that do not serve your health. Unplug the television. Uninstall unnecessary, time-sucking apps from your phone. This makes it harder to waste time on pointless activities.

This week just start with daily walking. Alternate day one and day two:

Day One
Six minutes of interval walking
Warm up with slow pace for two minutes
Walk at moderate pace for two minute.
Walk at slower pace for two minutes

Day Two
Six minutes of endurance walking.
Walk six minutes at a consistent, comfortable speed.

OR, If that is too easy for you try something a little longer:

Day One
Fifteen minutes of interval walking
Warm up with slow pace for two minutes
Walk at moderate pace for one minute.
Walk at slower pace for two minutes
Continue alternating for a total of 15 minutes

Day Two
Fifteen minutes of endurance walking.
Walk fifteen minutes at a consistent, comfortable speed.

Schedule it and track it. When are you going to get movement in? If you do not put it on your schedule, it is less likely to happen. What are you going to NOT do at that time? *Instead of watching tv after dinner I'm going to go for a walk.* Prioritize it!

Consistency and frequency are important. If walking is not your thing, do something else that you enjoy and look forward to doing every day or at least a few times a week. If you enjoy it, it will be easier to stick with. Walking with a friend can also help make it more enjoyable.

Nutrition

Remember the trap of moderation. If garbage, processed food is in your house, you will continually have to struggle not to eat it. The best way to avoid it is to remove it from your pantry and throw it away or give it away to someone whose health does not matter to you. Then stock your pantry and freezer with ingredients you can use for easy nutritious meals. Getting creative with substitutions is one easy way to start. If you are living with others who are not making changes, it can help to carve out an area for you so that you do not get distracted or tempted by foods you are eliminating.

Think of a meal you enjoy often. Pizza, burgers, tacos, pasta, chili? Is there a way to make it healthier? Making a meal at home ensures that what we are eating is healthy because we know what is in it. Less takeout usually means more nutrition. In home-cooked meals we can season and balance flavors to our individual preferences to make them mouthwatering. There is no need to overwhelm yourself with creating and learning all new recipes for every single meal. Start with some basics one at a time.

Food is part of our daily routine that we create rituals around. We often connect with other people in our life around food. When we share a meal with others, we focus more on what is on our plate. Eating while chatting with family or friends naturally helps us to slow down to eat and savor our meal.

The more we can be with our food instead of mindless shoveling, the easier it is to choose nutritious food. This week take time to slow down and be present with your food. Think about the flavors. Is it spicy, sour, sweet? Sitting down at a table to eat instead of eating over the kitchen sink, eating on the run or standing in the kitchen can help us pay more attention to our food. Slow down you pace, take smaller bites, and chew. Making mealtimes a "no devices" time is a good way to pay more attention to your food instead of being distracted by a phone, television, tablet, or computer.

For breakfast, oatmeal is a tried and-true healthy choice. Top it with whatever you like as long as you are not adding animal products

> *For breakfast, oatmeal is a tried-and-true healthy choice.*

like milk or butter. Keep it plant-based. Real maple syrup, raisins, chopped dates, hemp hearts, cinnamon, ginger, blueberries, bananas, apples and strawberries are all toppings I use often. Hashbrowns prepared in a no-stick pan or grill make a nice breakfast option, as does diced up fruit with dry toast.

Burgers are common on most menus in America. A simple substitution is a plant-based patty instead of a beef patty. The problem with most plant-based burgers at the store is that they have added oil. I find making them at home is the best way to get the nutrition I want. This week try making a batch of bean burgers.

Find a no-oil recipe that appeals to you or use this simple one:

Bean Burgers

1 15 ounce can of kidney beans (drain and mash in a mixing bowl with a fork)
½ cup cooked rice
½ cup oatmeal
1/8 cup tomato sauce
1 teaspoon Mrs. Dash or other no-salt all-purpose blend

1/8 teaspoon black pepper
½ teaspoon garlic powder

Stir all ingredients together in mixing bowl and chill for about 15 minutes. Form into patties and grill on no-stick griddle or skillet for 3-4 minutes on each side. If you want to make it even easier you can buy pre-cooked rice, or sometimes I use leftover mashed potatoes instead of rice.

I do not stress a lot over the bun except to see that it does not have milk or eggs in it. Once the patty has some usual toppings like tomato, lettuce, onion, pickles, ketchup, or mustard it is hard to recognize as a bean burger.

Pasta Marinara

Another meal that I feel is easy to substitute is a simple pasta dish. I usually use a jar of sauce from the store, - one with no oil when available. Then all you have to do is prepare whole grain (or gluten-free if needed) spaghetti noodles and heat the marinara sauce. If I have them on hand, I like to add some sliced mushrooms to the sauce when heating it. If you want to be super brave, add a handful or two of chopped spinach. Ladle the sauce over some noodles and you are done! This goes well with a simple side salad with oil-free dressing and a piece of rye bread (not greasy garlic bread).

As you begin to make substitutions in your regular meals you will start incorporating new recipes and noticing what cooking skills you are confident in and others that you would like to work on. Trust in the process. Gradually you will be more comfortable and confident with your ability to prepare delicious healthy meals.

Gradually you will be more comfortable and confident with your ability to prepare delicious healthy meals.

DON'T WAIT ANOTHER DAY CHANGE INSIDE

You will want to start stocking your pantry with foods you can keep on hand for a quick meal that tastes good. Some healthy ingredients to consider keeping on hand for these weeks and other meals are: frozen mushrooms, onions, peppers, stir-fry vegetables, rice, potatoes, corn, blueberries, strawberries, bananas, and green beans. In the pantry, consider stocking oil-free pasta sauce, whole grain pasta, rice, canned beans – black, garbanzo, pinto, oats, sweet potatoes, potatoes, squash, onions, and vinegars. In the refrigerator, some things I stock are pico de gallo, salsa, soy sauce, carrots, celery, apples, oranges, applesauce, and tofu. Keeping healthy foods on hand makes cooking healthy meals easier. When you decide what meals to create with these ingredients remember that when you choose to eat whole foods you are choosing to fuel your body with good nutrition.

Stress Reduction

Eliminating stress in your life can help with general health. Getting adequate sleep helps manage stress. This week concentrate on reducing stress with adequate sleep and connecting with your A-team.

Consider journaling, prayer, or meditation as a method of stress reduction. Limit interaction with toxic people in your life. Build relationships with your A-team. Exercise can also help with stress reduction. Notice what others around you do to reduce stress. Is it something you could try in your own life?

Consider journaling, prayer, or meditation as a method of stress reduction.

Have a great week!

CHAPTER NINE

Week Two

Seven days are done
Now keep up the momentum
Build on your progress

You made it this far! This week is very much the same as week one. This week is just adding gradual progression here and there. Consistent action with gradual progression allows us time to adapt and make changes. That is what it takes to get results.

Water

Same as last week, remember the general rule of thumb for staying hydrated is drink half your body weight in ounces of water. Add more for hot

If you are thirsty turn on the tap and enjoy rehydrating with warm, cold, or ice water.

weather, increased physical activity, or strenuous exercise. If you are thirsty turn on the tap and enjoy rehydrating with warm, cold, or ice water.

If it is helpful, continue using a graduated water bottle to track your fluid intake.

Sleep

Same as last week, remember general sleep recommendations are 8 hours per night. Children and teens may require more. Sleep for adults varies. Find what works for your body to feel rested.

Continue to do what it takes to create a clean, safe, quiet environment for sleep.

Develop a bedtime wind down routine. If you have not already, develop a bedtime wind down routine. This can be as simple as dimming lights and putting on soothing music. Pay attention to screen time before bed. Try to shut your electronics down an hour before you lay down. Sleep is required to recharge our body the same way we plug in our phone to recharge overnight.

Activity

Just because walking can be effortless does not mean it is not beneficial.

This week keep alternating day one and day two.

Only this week, as you do the endurance walk on day two, try to make it a meditation. Pay attention to your breath. Consider how your body feels. Feel your feet as they contact the ground. Think about how exercise can improve your mood, brain function and immune system. Remember each day you are building momentum. Each step you take leads to more action.

If walking is not your thing, consider the enjoyable activities you identified in Part One and do that instead. Make your activity something you have an ability for. If exercise satisfies you, you have a better chance of making room for it in your life.

> *Make your activity something you have an ability for.*

Day One
Six minutes of interval walking
Warm up with slow pace for two minutes
Walk at moderate pace for two minutes
Walk at slower pace for two minutes

Day Two
Six minutes of endurance walking.
Walk six minutes at a consistent, comfortable speed.

OR, If that is too easy for you try something a little longer:

Day One
Fifteen minutes of interval walking
Warm up with slow pace for two minutes
Walk at moderate pace for one minute
Walk at slower pace for two minutes
Continue alternating for a total of 15 minutes

Day Two
Fifteen minutes of endurance walking.
Walk fifteen minutes at a consistent, comfortable speed.

For bonus add a thirty second plank or 5-10 push-ups or bicep curls daily. Or add in other calisthenics such as 5-10 squats or try actively hanging on a bar or hanging rings.
Schedule it. Track it. Prioritize it!

Keep it short and sweet. Do not think it needs to be more than it does. Something is better than nothing. Unless you are training for a specific event, 30 minutes at a time is fine. Or even ten minutes at 3 different times in the day. It is good to have a plan A and a plan B. So if I plan to walk on my morning break and something comes up and I do not get to, I already have it set in my mind that I will walk later in the day at lunch or my afternoon break. Ideally, you stick with plan A and do not use plan B as a method of procrastination.

Keeping it simple and building gradually helps to avoid injury.

Also, remember keeping it simple and building gradually helps to avoid injury. Too often people try to do too much too quickly and end up hurting themselves. You will see results with consistent, progressive effort. I am a big believer in the saying, "Slow and steady wins the race."

Nutrition

As you continue to try new foods and recipes pay close attention to how it makes your body feel. Noticing positive changes can help you make better eating decisions. Being more aware of the food body connection is a thoughtful approach to eating, where you concentrate on nourishing your body and savoring what you eat, rather than, eating whatever is handy without paying attention to how it tastes or makes you feel.

As we go forward remember the pitfalls to avoid:

- Sugary drinks.
- Ultra-processed foods
- Added sugar
- Calorie dense foods (No added oil!)

- High fat foods (Limit animal products including meat, cheese, eggs, dairy, cheese, nuts, seeds, oils)

Try to protect your eating time so you are not eating on the run or during other tasks. How does it look? Smell? Taste? Eat slowly to give your brain time to register fullness. It is important to give your body enough calories to meet its needs so that you do not run out of energy. If you find yourself feeling hungry (not just bored) you probably are not eating enough calories. Good nutrition should *not* feel like a starvation diet. You can eat as much of the foods from week one and week two as you want until you feel satisfied.

Good nutrition should not feel like a starvation diet.

One way I have found to make nutritious food choices is to make less healthy food choices more difficult. For me, it starts at the store. If I do not buy processed food that is not healthy, then I do not have it in the pantry. If it is not in the house, I will not eat it. The more I eat nutritious food, the more momentum I have to pass up those fast-food chains that I used to go to when I was out of the house for the day. Sometimes I change my route so I do not have to pass places were I know I might be tempted to stop. If I know I am going to be gone from the house for long hours at a time I take food with me. Even if I forget to bring food, I remind myself that I am not going to starve in the four or five hours it takes me to get back home and fix a meal that I know is more nutritious and better for my body.

Make sure you are eating *enough* so you do not fizzle out!

Also think about timing. Ideally try to stop eating 2 hours before you go to bed. When you wake up if you are not hungry do not eat. Letting your body have 12 hours without food is fine. "Breakfast is the most important meal of the day" only applies IF you are hungry. When you are hungry eat. If you are not hungry, do not eat. Learn to pay attention to your body. When you do break your fast, whether it is first thing in the morning or more toward mid-day, the old saying, "Breakfast like a king, lunch like a prince, and dinner like a pauper," can be a good rule of thumb to put your body into a good rhythm. If you are out, keep in mind if you absolutely cannot find a plant-based meal to eat, remind yourself that you will not starve in the two hours until you get home. You can deal with a little bit of hunger from time to time without catastrophic results.

"Breakfast like a king, lunch like a prince, and dinner like a pauper, "

For week two I have selected some foods off the familiar food list and provided healthy version recipes for them.

Pancakes

The anti-carb campaign might have you feeling like pancakes are out of the question. Good news! They are fine if you do not make them using dairy or eggs and do not add butter or margarine or whipped cream (or any other fatty topping)

Eat your pancakes with real maple syrup – not the high fructose corn syrup kind. Better yet, top your pancakes with fresh fruit or frozen fruits heated into a warm compote. Sometimes I use applesauce as a topping.

Pancakes
1 cup flour
1 Tablespoon baking powder
1 cup non-dairy plant milk
2 Tablespoons water
1 teaspoon vanilla (optional)

1 teaspoon cinnamon (optional)
Mix all the ingredients together and **let rest 10 minutes**!

OR
Even Quicker Pancakes
Use a box mix that does not contain milk or eggs. Follow the box directions and sub in plant-milk or water for the liquid required, applesauce for any oil it may call for, and egg substitute for any egg (flax and water or other egg replacer).

Bread

Like pancakes, bread often gets a bad rap because it is a carb. Not all breads are created equal. The key is… do not eat breads made from refined sugars and refined white flour. Let your tastebuds get used to other kinds of whole grain or rye bread. This might take some time to get used to.

It is the carb-fat combo that gets us into trouble. A dry whole wheat bagel or bread topped with a fruit butter or applesauce is an okay choice. Ditch the cream cheese and butter. Even the nut butter spreads, hummus, and avocado spreads should be approached with caution because of their tendency to have high fat or added oils. Instead look for something lighter like a natural salsa, or a natural fruit spread or jam (that is not loaded with sugar).

As you can see, just in putting together week one and week two, you have a great variety of healthy, nutritious, breakfast options. You can usually find these types of foods when eating out. Sometimes it may mean ordering items a-la-carte. Sides like rice, steamed vegetables, plain baked potato, soup, or salad can come together to make a satisfying meal even at breakfast.

Fast Pizza

People who know me well know that pizza is one of my first loves in life. I remember Fridays in grade school. Those pre-packaged rectangular pizzas got me hooked and the rest is history! The sad part is that traditional American pizza is usually not a healthy choice. We already went over the cheese and dairy problems. The cheese alone sends pizza into a massive calorie trap. But I learned to fix it.

Step One: Buy or make a crust without oil and eggs in it and top it with a light layer of red marinara sauce or pizza sauce (one that is not loaded with oil).

Step Two: Add on the veggies of your choice. Green peppers, pineapple, onions, spinach, mushrooms, black olives, etc. I have even put on cooked diced potato or sweet potato. If you do not usually put veggies on your pizza this might be an adjustment.

If you find your pizza getting too soggy you can sauté the veggies in a tablespoon or two of water first to soften them and draw out some of the water, then use slotted spoon to lift them out and place on pizza.

Step Three: No cheese. What is pizza without the ooey gooey cheese, right? It is not the same, but it is also not as deadly, so it is a trade-off I am willing to accept. Not only that, but I also do not miss the cheese as much as I thought I would.

Cook for 8-10 minutes and you got a quick, healthy meal that you can feel good about.

Pasta Salad

Begin with choosing a whole grain pasta made *without* eggs. I like to use the bow-tie pasta, spirals, or penne for my pasta salad. You could also use veggie noodles such as zucchini noodles from the freezer section as an option.

Just like with our spaghetti, potatoes, breads, and salads, we must watch what we *put on* our pasta. Are you noticing a trend?

Here is a quick easy pasta salad:

Cook pasta as per package directions. Get a nice oil free dressing that you like (or make your own). While the pasta cooks, wash, and slice about a cup of cherry tomatoes. Drain the pasta (do not rinse under water unless it is a gluten-free pasta). While pasta is still hot, add a couple of handfuls of chopped spinach, about ¼ cup of dressing, and the cherry tomatoes. Stir and enjoy hot or cold.

You can add in chopped olives or chopped roasted red pepper for more color and flavor.

No added oil.

Remember that changing how you eat is not an easy task. You are going to be trying new recipes. Some

Take a second and give yourself a big round of applause.

you will like and others you will not. Your success will depend on your willingness to try new things and not to give up if you have a flop recipe.

Take a second and give yourself a big round of applause. You are taking it upon yourself to make changes in how you eat so that you have a healthy strong body. Way to go!

Burritos

Rice, like potatoes, gets plenty of bad press because of its carbohydrate content. Rice has been a staple for years especially in cultures that do not traditionally have chronic diseases. Healthy rice dishes make delicious meals that build a strong body.

This oil free Spanish rice can be added as a salad topping or used in burritos on top of beans with lettuce and salsa etc.

1 cup of brown rice
2 cups water
1 cup of tomato sauce
½ cup diced onion
1 teaspoon ground cumin
2 teaspoons chili powder
3-4 cloves minced garlic (or ¼ teaspoon garlic powder)

Put all ingredients together in a small pot or rice cooker. Bring to a boil or set cooker. Cook until liquid is absorbed. Fluff with fork and let rest about 5 minutes prior to serving. Salt and pepper to taste.

Spanish rice will work perfect in a bean burrito. If you prefer, you can use *plain* cooked brown rice. Drain and mash a can of black beans and spread some on the burrito shell, top with cooked rice and one or more of these other options: corn, salsa, lettuce, guacamole – skip the cheese and sour cream. It is easy, fast, and nutritious.

Another burrito I like to make looks like this:

Sauté a package of frozen pepper onion mixture in a few tablespoons of water and add some sliced mushrooms – cook 3-4 minutes in a skillet until hot. Add a can of drained and rinsed pinto beans and about a cup of cooked rice. Then, if you are lucky enough to have it in a store near you, add a half a package of Frontera Classic Fajita Skillet Sauce with Chipotle & Lime. This is so easy and fast it feels like cheating!

This is so easy and fast it feels like cheating!

Make a double batch and store the leftovers in the fridge for a quick grab and go meal.

Stew

Stew is also super-fast and good to make once or twice a week to have as a grab and go meal. Not to mention, one-pot stews are an easy way to prepare a meal without getting every pot and utensil in the kitchen dirty.

Here is a simple formula for a one-pot stew:
Over medium heat in a pot, or in a crock pot add a base flavor such as garlic, onions, and ginger.
Add chopped veggies.
Add base liquids such as a tomato product/sauce or diced or low salt vegetable stock. Or use water.
Add cooked grains or beans of your choice.
Season with acids, spices, and herbs.
In a few hours you will have a delightful stew to eat with salads & sandwiches.

Try this:
1 onion, diced
3 cloves of garlic, minced
1 teaspoon ginger, minced
2 stalks of celery, diced
2 carrots, diced
1 green bell pepper, diced
1 red bell pepper, diced
2 cups diced potatoes
2 cans cannellini beans, drained and rinsed
2 cups tomato sauce
2 cups low sodium vegetable broth
3 cups water
1 tablespoon parsley flakes
1 tablespoon low sodium soy sauce
1 teaspoon basil

1 teaspoon oregano
1/8 teaspoon crushed red pepper
1/4 cup brown rice
3 handfuls of chopped spinach

Place ingredients except the rice and spinach in a crock pot turn on low and let cook 4-6 hours.

OR soften onion, celery, carrot, and bell pepper in a soup pot 5-7 minutes on medium heat with about ½ cup of water. Add remaining ingredients except the rice & spinach and cook for about an hour over low heat stirring as needed.

When veggies are softened, add rice and spinach and cook additional 5 minutes.

You can use other cooked grains such as quinoa, bulgur, or millet & you can use other beans such as garbanzo beans instead of white. Instead of baby potatoes – you can use whatever you have.

For dessert week two we have:

Pumpkin Pie

Mix:
2 tablespoons cornstarch
2 teaspoons cinnamon
2 teaspoons baking powder
½ cup brown sugar
½ cup all-purpose flour
½ teaspoon nutmeg
½ teaspoon ground ginger
½ teaspoon cardamon
1/8 teaspoon salt

In a separate large bowl combine:
½ cup silken tofu (I have used soft, but silken is better)
1 ½ cups almond milk
1 teaspoon of vanilla
2 cups of pumpkin pure pumpkin (not pumpkin pie mix)

Mix the dry ingredients into the wet and pour into a parchment paper lined 9" pie pan or a vegan pie crust.

Cook for 1 hour at 350 degrees.

Usually, I just cook it using the parchment paper without a crust. It takes 30-60 minutes or so to set up as it cools. I store it in the fridge, and I usually eat the leftovers cold.

Find what works for you! Just remember - No eggs. No dairy. No whipped cream topping.

Other pies you can learn to make without dairy, eggs, or oils are chocolate banana pie and apple pie.

Sorbet

Sorbet is a nice frozen dessert that does not have any fat or cholesterol. You can buy it at the grocery store – check the label! Or you can use this recipe for Strawberry Lemon Sorbet:

1 cup of water
1/8 cup of sugar
1 Tablespoon of lemon juice
1 pound of frozen unsweetened strawberries

Allow strawberries to thaw at room temperature for about 5 minutes.

In a food processor or high-speed blender, combine all ingredients in the order listed. Blend until smooth. Eat it right away or freeze it in serving size containers until ready to serve.

Another popular frozen fruit dessert is "nice" cream with frozen bananas.

Putting good nutrition together with other lifestyle modifications such as adequate sleep, regular fitness activity, and stress management can help prevent & treat disease. Remember the purpose of taking time to learn new recipes is to support your health. New ways of preparing and thinking about your food are worth the effort it takes to learn.

Stress Reduction

Eliminating stress in your life can help with general health. Getting adequate sleep helps manage stress. This week continue to reduce stress with adequate sleep and connecting with your A-team. At the same time, if you have not already, pick another stress reduction technique to try. My wake-up routine and my bedtime routine are good places for sitting in meditation, journaling, or prayer. Lunch time also works well for me.

The important thing is to just start somewhere. Before I began meditating, I thought it was all about sitting with my eyes closed and emptying my mind. As I began to practice meditation, I have found that it is something I can do even while running or emptying the dishwasher. Pick an activity that you can do on autopilot and practice being more aware of your body, movement, and surroundings as you do it. Count the dishes as you put them away. Notice how the silverware feels in your hand. Be in the moment as you complete the task. This is a way to quiet our racing minds and reduce the stress that comes with busy-ness. This week look for opportunities in your day to slow down and be present. Of course, traditional sitting meditation and stillness with prayer are helpful in reducing stress too. Quiet journaling and allowing your mind to sift through thoughts can be good stress relief.

Taking a shower can be a daily routine that turns into meditation. You choose your thoughts throughout your day. You can choose to listen to relaxing music and really pay attention to the instruments and notes you hear. Guided imagery is another technique that helps to reduce stress.

As you try different methods to be present and aware in the moment you will find more than one technique that you can incorporate into your day. Do not limit what meditation looks like. There is more than one way to practice. Allowing yourself to explore different techniques will make it easier to find one with which you can stick. Resist the urge to get tripped up on future thinking. Find what works for today and take it one day at a time.

> *Resist the urge to get tripped up on future thinking.*

Have a great week!

CHAPTER TEN

Week Three

One day at a time
The foundation is stronger
As weeks turn to months

Before we move into week three let us recap on the healthy habits we have been working on.

- More water to keep us hydrated (and less high calorie sugary/salty drinks)
- Get proper rest with adequate sleep time of 7-8 hours per night
- Be active but do not overdo it. Do not underestimate low level work. Regular exercise of at least 4 days per week – as natural as walking.
- Eat whole food plant-based nutrition avoiding animal products, processed foods, and added oils therefore low in sugar, salt, and fat (avoiding alcohol, tobacco, and drugs). Set yourself up for success by planning so you are not relying on willpower alone.
- Nurture our minds and relationships

- Stress reduction using any or all: exercise, meditation, prayer, mindfulness, journaling.
- Strive to eliminate smoking, alcohol, and drugs. Remember the notion of moderation only makes it more difficult to quit because continually having to rely on willpower in the face of too many choices may end up leaving us frustrated and/or emotional.

As we continue to practice these healthy habits we move from destruction of our health with processed food, sedentary life, drama, and stress, to supporting our health with good nutrition, decreased stress, exercise, being present in each moment, and healthy, supportive relationships.

Water

Continue with drinking water daily. Some research suggests the human body is up to 60% water. The brain and heart are over 70% water, and the lungs are estimated to be as high as over 80% water. Muscle and kidneys are near 80% as well. Even bones are estimated to be about 30% water. The largest organ is our skin, and it is over 60% water. We can appreciate our body and take care of it simply by giving it the water it needs.

We can appreciate our body and take care of it simply by giving it the water it needs.

If you want to step it up a notch this week, or if you are getting bored with plain water. Try adding some flavor to your water. You can do this with fruits like lemon, lime, orange, strawberries, or grapes. Consider using cranberry concentrate, pineapple juice, or even flavor drops or powders (read the labels!) to add some flavor to your water.

Sleep

Choose to be aware of your surroundings with meditation or prayer before bed, remember that what we ponder before bed sticks with us while we sleep. Information we feed our mind can have impact on our daily life and our sleep. Harness the good and block the bad. What we read, watch, and listen to before bed stays with us through the night and into the following days even after we turn it off.

Thankfulness makes us happy strengthening our heart and immune system. This makes bedtime a prime time to acknowledge our thoughts with meditation, prayer, or journaling to tap into an attitude of gratitude. Consider how you love yourself and others. Think about what you are doing to care for your body. Think about what you can do for other people in your life and how they help to care for you.

Activity

Take a walk. As you walk, think about the things in your life you are thankful for. Sometimes when I am exercising, I focus on being grateful that I am able to do whatever exercise I am doing to prevent muscle loss, decrease my risk for disease, build an appetite, and/or increase energy levels.

Think about the things in your life you are thankful for.

Another day take a walk outdoors if possible. Some research indicates time in nature can boost our happiness and make us increase our positivity. In addition to walking, simple calisthenics can do wonders for our body.

While activity is important, do not let it take the front seat to good nutrition. It does not matter how much you exercise if you are eating the wrong food. Do not mess up on the food. "Abs are made in the kitchen!"

Nutrition

Think: *Am I hungry? What does my body need?*

Soup in a blender, smoothies in a blender, and batch cooking for bowl building and meal planning can help us save time while still getting good nutrition.

If you have not already, start a list of meals you have been trying and making that are whole food plant-based. Include any foods that were already in your meal rotation prior to any recent new meals. Do you eat fresh fruit - like apples, bananas, and grapes,- toast, oatmeal, peanut butter and jelly, salads, baked potatoes, vegetables, bean burritos, tacos, stir-fry, soups, bean chili, or mashed potatoes?

What soup recipes have you found that you enjoy?

Have you had any new sandwiches or pizza that has worked for you? Need help building your list?

Here are some of my favorite, familiar foods:

Oatmeal, Bran Flakes with non-dairy plant milk, bran muffins, pancakes, cinnamon rolls, hashbrowns, waffles, grits, bagels, toast, fruit, smoothies, tofu scramble, burritos

Bean soup, tacos, bean or mushroom burgers, lentil sloppy joe, pasta salad, potato salad, green salads, pizza (without dairy cheese), vegetable soup, minestrone soup, burritos

Spaghetti, veggie lasagna, burritos, stew, stir-fry, sushi, cabbage rolls, stuffed peppers, tex-mex pasta, "cheesy" broccoli pasta, mac and cheese, fajitas, bean chili, burritos, steamed or roasted vegetables, baked potato or rice with plant-based toppings

Bowl building: cook rice in a large batch and freeze any extra. Add shredded carrots, sprouts, beans, spinach, or kale, and/or sauteed mushrooms.

Rice pudding, chocolate pudding, peach crisp, apple crisp, carrot cake, pumpkin pie, pumpkin pudding, peach pie, fruit, sorbet

As you try new recipes you will learn which ones are your favorites. These are ones you might consider preparing a double batch of so there is always something easy to grab from the refrigerator or freezer on busy days. You will begin to realize that, with a little planning, cooking seven days a week is optional.

Meat Loaf

Before I began eating plant-based nutrition meat loaf was one of the meals I had in rotation. After trying a few recipes, I have found a couple that I like. This one reminds me of Thanksgiving stuffing.

Oat, Tofu, and Lentil Loaf

1½ cups chopped celery
¾ cup onion
3 cloves garlic, minced
10 ounces firm tofu, pressed & drained
¼ cup finely chopped walnuts
½ cup cooked lentils
1 ¼ cup oats
3 Tablespoons soy sauce
2 Tablespoons BBQ sauce
1 Tablespoon Dijon mustard
1 Tablespoon dried parsley
1 teaspoon thyme

½ teaspoon sage
½ teaspoon rosemary

Saute celery & onion in water until softened. Add garlic and saute about 1 more minute. Cool.
Mash tofu in a large bowl. Stir in walnuts, lentils, and oats. Mix remaining ingredients in a small bowl and then stir into tofu mixture. Add in cooled celery & onion.
Spoon mixture into parchment lined loaf pan & press lightly. Top with an optional light layer of additional BBQ sauce, then bake at 375 degrees for one hour or until cake tester or toothpick comes out clean. I enjoy this with mashed potatoes and gravy, green beans, and cranberry sauce. It also makes good leftovers the next day on a sandwich.
Another recipe to consider trying that makes good leftovers is the following pasta dish.

Tex-Mex Pasta

1 sliced zucchini
1 ½ cups frozen corn
3-4 cloves of garlic
1 teaspoon oregano
1 15 ounce can of black beans
1 15 ounce can low salt diced tomatoes
2 cups spinach, chopped
Fresh basil chopped
Salt and pepper to taste
4 ounces penne pasta cooked according to package directions

Saute zucchini, corn, garlic, oregano in a skillet until tender.
Add black beans and tomatoes
Add cooked penne and spinach. Fold together over medium heat until spinach is wilted.

Stress Reduction

I talk about your A-team a lot and how they support you. This week keep in mind how your relationship adds to *their* life. Be there for them to if they need help or to cheer them in a success. A group of friends are not just about leaning on each other through challenges, but they are also there to celebrate triumphs, milestones, and the joys of life. This week consider what you contribute to your group.

To help you reap the benefits of relationships we need regular social time. Schedule in a phone call or video call at the very least with your close friends so that you keep in touch. A lunch date, dinner date or walking date in person is even better. Either way, the more important thing is consistent connection to help strengthen your relationships. Surrounding yourself with people who have the same values can help you feel supported and hold you accountable which also makes us less stressed. As we are more connected, we increase our gratitude, kindness, and compassion as well. Not to mention it gives us more opportunity to laugh and smile which releases serotonin to lift our mood.

> *This week consider what you contribute to your group.*

This week you could also designate a day of gratitude where you will focus only on one thing: being grateful.

Hobbies outside of exercise can also help reduce stress and give us a sense of purpose. Hobbies are a fun reason to get out of bed in the morning. Gardening, knitting, spending time with pets, woodworking, - whatever it is that excites you is worth pursuing for the stress relief it brings. Other people find it therapeutic to take care of extended family or volunteering within their community. So long as it is something that feels fulfilling to you (and is not destructive to others), that's what hobbies are all about.

Pick something genuine to who you are.

Not The End.

This is not the end. The beginning is the end and the end is the beginning. Life goes around in one big circle. Round and round we go as we grow and change. Changes in our lifestyle habits have a ripple effect in our own life. As we improve the health of our physical body, we are also nourishing our soul.

We are expanding as the circles go out around us.

Our hope for better health is our confidence that our desires and expectations are possible. That hope ripples out into our community. Living authentic lives with joy and focus help us to overcome our vices and live in virtue as much as we can. Attempting to live in virtue is messy and we will never be perfect at it.

Changing lifestyle habits requires patience and humility. We make mistakes. We all can own our hypocrisy and get up and try again tomorrow. Our patience and humility ripple out in circles into the world.

Living in virtue is living in generosity, love, forgiveness, and friendship. These virtues are food from heaven better than any we have here on Earth. This is the food that satisfies our hungry hearts, so we do not become weak in life.

Your big, delicious life is meant to be lived in Whole with those around you. Our body is just getting us through as we go through the ups and downs of life. Our soul goes beyond our physical limitations. Our body and soul work together. This is what we are sending out.

Take care of your body and you are caring for your soul.

You can have the quality of life and health you were created to have. Put in the work today that you want to send out in ripples to expand and circle the world.

The Beginning.

Acknowledgements

Thanks be to God for all the blessings bestowed on me in this life, including the opportunity to author this book. I appreciate the serendipitous moments along the journey with people, circumstances, and information provided just when I was in need. People surrounded and supported me as I planned for and drafted this book. I could not have completed it without those of you who listened to my vision, had patience with me during the writing process, and offered feedback, editing, extra time, and proofreading. Thank you for believing in me, encouraging me, and inspiring me! You know who you are. Special thanks to Glenn, Judith, Jarod, Zechariah, Samantha, Alexander, Leila, Adam, Mrs. T, Jacob, Michael, Jennifer, Jamie, Tanisha, Marissa, Josh, Jessica, Teri, Debbie, Jessabelle, and all the wonderful people at AAE who gave me freedom to allow the book to evolve as needed, and all my helpers at JETLAUNCH who made it look presentable. You rock!

About the Author

Catherine Hirsch is a registered nurse who proclaims the message: with God's help lifestyle medicine can heal our body, restore our spirit, and overcome injustice in our world. Catherine has been certified in plant-based nutrition since 2019, a plant-based culinary school graduate since 2020, and is in the process of becoming a certified yoga instructor. Since discovering the benefits of lifestyle medicine, she has made it her mission to bring its healing effects to her clients and friends. She resides with her family in southern Ohio. To connect go to: DontWaitChangeInside.com

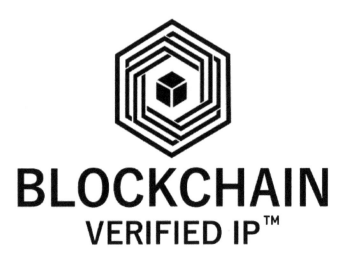

BLOCKCHAIN
VERIFIED IP™

Powered by Easy IP™

Ingram Content Group UK Ltd.
Milton Keynes UK
UKHW021603110723
424927UK00015B/453